ROUTLEDGE LIBRARY EDITIONS:
JAPAN

HEALTH CARE IN JAPAN

HEALTH CARE IN JAPAN

MARGARET POWELL
AND MASAHIRA ANESAKI

Volume 79

Routledge
Taylor & Francis Group
LONDON AND NEW YORK

First published in 1990

This edition first published in 2011
by Routledge
4 Park Square, Milton Park, Abingdon, Oxon OX14 4RN
605 Third Avenue, New York, NY 10017

Routledge is an imprint of the Taylor & Francis Group, an informa business

British Library Cataloguing in Publication Data
A catalogue record for this book is available from the British Library

ISBN 13: 978-0-415-56498-4 (Set)
eISBN 13: 978-0-203-84317-8 (Set)
ISBN 13: 978-0-415-59541-4 (Volume 79) (hbk)
eISBN 13: 978-0-203-84128-0 (Volume 79)

Health Care in Japan

Margaret Powell and Masahira Anesaki

ROUTLEDGE
London and New York

First published in 1990
by Routledge
11 New Fetter Lane, London EC4P 4EE

Simultaneously published in the USA and Canada
by Routledge
a division of Routledge, Chapman and Hall, Inc.
29 West 35th Street, New York, NY 10001

Typeset by Mayhew Typesetting, Bristol
Printed and bound in Great Britain by
Biddles Ltd, Guildford and King's Lynn

British Library Cataloguing in Publication Data

Powell, Margaret, *1947–*
Health care in Japan.
1. Japan. Health services
I. Title II. Anesaki, Masahira, *1936–*
362.1'0952

Library of Congress Cataloging in Publication Data

Powell, Margaret, 1947–
Health care in Japan/Margaret Powell and Masahira Anesaki.
p. cm.
Bibliography: p.
Includes index.
1. Medical care – Japan. 2. Public health – Japan. I. Anesaki, Masahira, 1936– . II. Title.
[DNLM: 1. Delivery of Health Care – Japan. W 84 JJ3 P8h]
RA531.P68 1989
362.1'0952 – dc20
DNLM/DLC
for Library of Congress 89-10161
CIP

ISBN 0-415-00610-4

Contents

Chapter one

Introduction

In 1986 Japan numbered among her 119 million citizens some 1,851 people who were over 100 years old. Among this elite group women outnumbered men by a ratio of four to one; until February 1986 the honour of being the world's oldest reliably documented citizen fell on the shoulders of a 120-year-old man called Shigechiyo Izumi, a resident of southern Japan whose birthday was recorded as 29 June 1865 and who attributed his longevity to a daily drink of 'shochu' (rice spirit) and leaving things up to Buddha.

The first life-table for Japan covered the years 1891 to 1898 and showed that a Japanese male born during those years could expect to live for just over 42 years; a Japanese female born at the same time had a couple of years' edge and could therefore expect to reach 44 years of age. After the Second World War, in 1947, both sexes had gained an additional ten years. By 1985 life expectancy was just under 81 years for Japanese women and 75 years for men. For almost a decade Japan has been ranked in the top five countries on this indicator of health status.

In the past hundred years too, striking gains have been made in the infant mortality rate, another widely accepted measure of social health and well-being. For every one hundred babies born in 1915, fifteen would die in their first year of life. The infant mortality rate has improved spectacularly during the century and in 1986 had reached a low of 5.5 per 1,000 live births, placing Japan in the number one position in the world.[1] The crude death-rate for the country has declined considerably, from 25.4 per 1,000 in 1920 to 6.2 per 1,000 in 1983. It is clear on the evidence of such statistics that Japan has equalled and often surpassed other developed countries in the gains she has made in the standard measures used to assess a nation's health status.

At the same time however, Japan appears well down the list in any international league table covering expenditure on health care. In common with developed and developing countries alike Japan has witnessed considerable growth in national expenditure on health care services since the end of the Second World War; the rate of increase in spending was especially marked during the 1960s and 1970s. The proportion of gross national product (GNP) devoted to health rose from 3 per cent in 1960 to 6.7 per cent in 1983,[2] an increase which has caused concern in the country. By comparison with other developed countries which enjoy the same high health status, Japan's official expenditure is in fact extremely low. The USA spent rather more than 10 per cent of GNP on health care in 1983, up from 5.3 per cent in 1960; France and Sweden each spent more than 9 per cent in 1983. In its survey of health care spending among member countries the Organization for Economic Co-operation and Development (OECD) presented figures which show that of twenty-three countries only seven countries (Spain, Greece, Luxembourg, New Zealand, Portugal, Belgium, and the United Kingdom) devoted the same or a smaller proportion of GNP to health expenditure as Japan in 1982. A superficial look at the available statistical data presents therefore a puzzling and seemingly paradoxical picture for Japan: it has remarkably good health indices and what seems to be an extremely low burden of health costs.

At first sight then the Japanese scenario seems to lend some weight to the arguments of a growing number of critics of the organized health services who consider that the level of spending on health care *per se*, and specifically on medical services, seems to bear scant relationship to the quality of health consequently enjoyed, or not as the case may be, by the recipients of care. More has not necessarily meant better.

We have written this book in order to provide a description of the historical development, the social, political, and cultural factors which have been instrumental in producing the system for the provision of health care in Japan today. In gathering together information and data to provide an up-to-date review of the principal features of the Japanese health care system we have also tried to probe behind the obvious, to throw some light on some problematic issues in the area of health and medical services in this country and to present a critical examination of some of the approaches which are being developed in order to solve acknowledged problems in the health system.

There are some straightforward questions about health care in Japan which we consider are not adequately covered by the existing and enormous range of publications about Japan. We shall therefore present some descriptive information designed to answer a number of very obvious questions. In population size Japan ranks as the seventh largest country in the world and her economy is the third largest in the world: how does this prosperous, crowded island nation care for her sick? What proportion of the nation's wealth is allocated to health and welfare services? How is the provision of health care financed? Does the individual have to pay for services and treatment and if so how is payment made? Is there a health insurance system and how is it structured? Japan has acquired a dazzling reputation for her industrial management practices; are the same principles employed in the organization and management of her health care services? If so are these principles appropriate? Are Japanese health services efficient and effective or is there scope for improvement? What are the gaps in present services? Who formulates health policy? Who are the interested parties in the policy formulation process and whose interests do they represent? How are doctors trained in Japan? Who is responsible for monitoring standards of medical practice? How are doctors remunerated? Can patients exercise freedom of choice in selecting a doctor or hospital? How do patients view the services and care that is provided? Are their views taken into account by policy-makers and service-providers?

In Japan as in other developed countries economic progress and development have resulted in dramatic improvements in living standards. Together with social and economic progress have come substantial changes in patterns of morbidity and mortality; the incidence and prevalence of infectious diseases have declined and there has been an increase in the prevalence of the chronic degenerative diseases which are more complex in their aetiology and treatment.

For Japan as elsewhere the accuracy and reliability of official data on health expenditure cannot be guaranteed; nor can official statistics which are necessarily compiled for public consumption and international comparison be fully equated with the total costs of care, which include the less quantifiable social and personal costs of ill-health. The seemingly low level of health care costs in Japan is the result partly of the way the system is organized and financed and this in turn has evolved over a considerable period of time. The system has proved to be adequate in the past because a complex interweaving of social and cultural factors has to some extent depressed the burden of costs to the state; there is concern that changes in these factors will be such that the system will not be capable of continuing to function with anything like the same degree of effectiveness as it has to date. Social and cultural patterns have therefore had a protective effect and have helped to defray the real increase in costs which should have been taking place. As Japan approaches the end of the twentieth century social and cultural changes will be coupled with dramatic demographic and economic developments which together will necessitate substantial amendments to the structure of the Japanese health care system which, like the Japanese economy, seems to have enjoyed only runaway success.

Japan as Number One is the cliché often favoured in describing the economic giant which is Japan today. A legion of publications has documented, debated, and puzzled over the factors which have been instrumental in Japan's economic achievements over the past forty years. 'From the rubble of defeat Japan has built an economy that is an inspiration to the developing world and a formidable competitor for the Industrial world.'[3] Any first-time visitor to Japan is forcefully struck by the visible signs of prosperity. Impressions are further reinforced by reference to consumer surveys and opinion polls, which regularly and consistently record that a high proportion of the citizens of Japan consider themselves to be happy, comfortable, and much better off than their parents were. An astonishing 90 per cent moreover hold themselves to be members of the middle class. Looking beyond the smartly turned out shopping crowds and the beautiful window displays of highly expensive goods there are details of Japanese life-styles and the environment which the Japanese too are beginning to express doubts about. At the same time as appreciating the undoubted material benefits and improvements which are the demonstrable results of some forty years of concentration on economic investment and growth many Japanese are beginning to look more searchingly at their environment, to ask some telling questions about their society, and its qualitative aspects.

The social services are notoriously under-developed for a country of such obvious wealth and which espouses egalitarian principles. The official neglect of social welfare (including health) programmes has been possible because traditional values and customs have meant that state provisions were held to be either unnecessary or unwanted by the community. Japan is frequently described as having a highly developed sense of group consciousness together with strong feelings of responsibility for members of the group. The group can encompass a number of entities – the family, village, city neighbourhood, office section, or factory work unit. The family is the foremost group to which allegiance is required and the family in turn has traditionally looked after its members. Even though there has been some loosening of traditional family ties and responsibility these remain, in comparison with standards prevailing in the west, demonstrably strong. While the majority, some 60 per cent, of households now consist of nuclear family units, an average of 50 per cent of all elderly people aged 65 and over still live with their children.[4] A survey in the Metropolitan Tokyo area in 1985[5] demonstrated that 55 per cent of people over 65 years of age lived with their children or other family members; 29 per cent with their spouse only and 14 per cent were living alone. The health and social services provided by the state in Japan to date have been acceptable because they fitted in with the thinking and customs of the Japanese population. The idea that society at large rather than the immediate family group has a responsibility for elderly and sick people may, for example, nowadays appear to have official endorsement but in actuality the family remains primarily responsible for the care and welfare of its sick and elderly members. State provision of services and facilities lags behind those of other developed nations and the state has been satisfied to finance a level of provision which is the minimum acceptable, a safety net approach. The system of health and medical care has also reflected the preferences of the principal providers of services, namely the medical profession, who have likewise capitalized on cultural values to preserve and continue the status quo. There is some evidence of growing consumer dissatisfaction with the health services offered and some medical practitioners and specialists are raising questions for debate because of concern about the costs of providing services for a larger number of elderly people in a society which will not be able to continue to depend on family supports. The relative and absolute increase in the numbers of elderly people is occurring moreover at the same time as the relative size of the working population is decreasing; a smaller number of people will therefore have to support the increasing financial burden. People aged 65 and over constituted 9 per cent of the total population in 1983 and will make up 17 per cent of the population in 2005.[6] All the developed industrial nations have experienced declines in birth-rates and death-rates, leading to a shift to an ageing population, and Japan is no exception. However the pace at which this transition is happening in Japan is exceptionally rapid; this demographic shift, which occurred over a period of sixty years in the United Kingdom, is taking place within a span of twenty years in Japan. In 1982 the costs of medical care for people aged 65 and over were 39 per cent of in-patient costs and 28 per cent of out-patient costs. More than a third of the total medical care costs bill went on services for elderly patients.[7] Japan has to evaluate how she can best provide the appropriate type of care for her elderly population in the years to come.

At the same time as coping with a greater burden of welfare spending Japan will be running an economy projected to be marked by a period of reduced growth.[8] Between 1955 and 1973 Japan's average annual economic growth rate was 9.5 per cent. Since the first oil crisis of 1973 Japan's growth rate has slowed and between 1976 and 1980 real GNP growth rates averaged 5.1 per cent. Japan, like her counterparts in Europe, will be compelled to find ways of maintaining an acceptable level of spending on social welfare programmes in balance with national finances. Whether, and indeed if the present system of health and medical services is capable of achieving an acceptable balance of care is a major issue among health services specialists in Japan today. This will be one of the questions we will look at as we examine various aspects of medical care.

Research studies and publications about Japan have encompassed a wide range of subjects, some of which have been more intensively covered than others. As the British historian G.B. Sansom noted in his Foreword to Edwin Reischauer's classic study *Japan: Past and Present* (first published in 1946), 'Few countries have been more copiously described than Japan and perhaps few have been less thoroughly understood'.[9] In the forty years since those words were written the volume of publications has taken on the scale and dynamism of what the Japanese might aptly call a 'tsunami' or tidal wave.

The umbrella term 'Japanese studies' includes a number of broad categories: history, including general chronological accounts of life in Japan from the earliest times up to the present; studies of particular features of Japanese history such as feudalism, courtly life, the role of the samurai; impressions of Japan and travellers' tales, all make immensely fascinating reading. Language and literature studies include the translation of works of Japanese literature; in culture and the arts subjects discussed are drama, Kabuki and Noh, ceramics, religion and philosophy, 'sumie' (ink painting), and woodblock prints. In the social sciences the study of politics has featured predominantly and especially so since the Meiji Restoration of 1868, which saw the opening up of the country after more than two hundred years of deliberately self-imposed isolation. Japan's foreign policy and foreign relations have been a natural choice for study and analysis. There have been comprehensive and illuminating studies of Japan's transformation from a feudalistic agricultural society to one of the world's leading industrial powers.

Japan's economic success story since the end of the Second World War has been steadily documented and monitored over the years; its continuing economic success in the late 1970s and early 1980s, a time moreover when other major economies have faltered, has if anything prompted an even greater number of observers, pundits and commentators to publish their thoughts and views on what keeps 'Japan Inc.' rolling along so nicely. Within the broad field of the social sciences, however, the focus of interest has been largely on specific subject matter closely related to or which can throw light on factors contributing to Japan's economic achievements. In the majority of studies the overall tone has been positively sycophantic and most writers have written admiringly about what has been achieved by a small island nation so lacking in natural resources. This admiring tone is however being replaced by more critical views; a number of publications have started to question the social bases of Japan's economy. It is perhaps significant that social administration, social welfare, and social policy have been relatively neglected areas of research. The seeming lack of interest in social welfare to some extent reflects a relative lack of importance within Japan herself in the last thirty to forty years; another interpretation might be that these areas have not impinged in any obvious fashion on the economic bases of so many of the world's major powers as has Japan's manifest ability to produce and sell effectively such enormous numbers of high-quality cars, motorcycles, cameras, electronic components equipment, and consumer goods. It has been far more critical for western nations to be able to fathom out and understand how Japan organizes and manages her trade and industry than how she provides pensions for her retired, and organizes health care for her sick. The growing interest in social welfare and social policy in Japan among western specialists to some extent has paralleled a growing concern among the Japanese themselves about provisions for the less able members of her materialistically successful society.

The Japanese health and medical services have not been widely studied or evaluated by international specialists but interest, quite rightly, is growing. Abel-Smith emphasizes the positive value of acquiring information and understanding about the organization and financing of health services in different countries.[10] He notes too that his descriptions of other systems are limited by the availability of literature in the English language. In many publications in the field of comparative health studies it is quite singular that Japan is inevitably included in the statistical tables; passing references are made to her considerable achievements in lowering mortality and infant mortality rates and the low level of expenditure on health care as a percentage of GNP may be noted. Further discussion or elaboration of the statistics is usually very limited and, given the lack of reference materials, this is not surprising.

The growing interest in how countries organize, finance, and deliver their health services is founded in a number of reasons. Expenditure on health services has risen dramatically in all countries in the past thirty years; much of the expansion in the health services of developed countries took place in the 1960s and 1970s when the economic climate was conducive to greater investment in health care and in the development and promotion of improved therapies and technology which were becoming available. Many countries subsequently encountered serious health care financing problems in the late 1970s and early 1980s as they were compelled to come to terms with economic recession necessitating reductions in the level of expenditure on health services. The expansion of services and improved access to them together with the spread of new technologies and therapies all contributed to rising public expectations about the outcome of medical care and to higher utilization of services. At the same time, however, changing patterns of morbidity were the source of concern about the ability of medical science to provide the right kind of care and treatment. Demographic changes contributed further to organizational and financial problems.

There are many different systems of health service delivery in the world today; all countries have developed either consciously or by default, a pattern of health service organization which is in keeping with their culture, values, political system, and economic status. While individuality and differences among health systems will undoubtedly continue, these diverse systems none the less share some similarities, more than might at first be expected.

To a greater or lesser extent the trend in each country has been for the government to take greater responsibility and control in the financing and organization of health services. Roemer describes this development in some detail noting, 'Collectivisation has been applied both to the systems of economic support for health services and to the patterns of provisions for delivery of those services. The effect has been to make more health services available to more people.'[11]

Access to health services is widely available in the developed countries of the world and is on the whole assured; such access remains problematic in many developing countries. As we have noted, however, there is growing concern in many developed countries about the appropriateness of health service provisions to the health care needs of the population. The emphasis on medical care and the increasing reliance on new technology have contributed to the cost spiral without always achieving the expected outcomes of improved health care and health status. Duplication and misuse of high-cost resources are doubly wasteful at a time when demographic and social conditions require a more careful use of limited resources.

Many countries have been forced to review the underlying philosophy of their health policies and have had to implement often controversial changes in patterns of provision in order to ensure that equitable access to the best quality care is possible while costs are at the same time contained. Despite some similarities in policy the specific programme solutions chosen offer great variety; the experience of one country cannot be transferred lock, stock, and barrel to another. Each nation's values and traditions are such that simple acceptance of systems grounded in completely different cultural soil is unpalatable.

However as long as the problems retain some common features it is only sensible and reasonable to acquire and share information about them. Knowledge of the experiences of other countries in tackling the same or similar difficulties may be illuminating even if it only helps in an assessment of which solutions are impracticable. If we know something of how other countries organize, finance, and deliver their health services we also begin to acquire some insight into the social traditions and prevailing values of that country. What kinds of problems have been encountered and what have been the solutions tried? Which approaches have been successful and which have failed dismally? What factors have been critical in the success or failure of a particular programme? Can a particularly successful solution be adopted for use elsewhere or will it work only if it is adapted and used in a modified form? Because these common problems are becoming more critical the search for solutions is taking on a degree of urgency and experience elsewhere cannot sensibly be ignored but can rather offer valid lessons and alternatives.

It is our intention to provide as comprehensive and lucid an account of the health care delivery system in Japan today as is possible within the confines of a single text. To do this we have necessarily had to approach the selection of subject matter and issues for discussion with some circumspection. The reader who knows nothing about health care in Japan should find the descriptive and factual information up to date and sufficiently detailed enough to obtain a broad understanding of the essentials; we do not presume to pursue satisfactorily all the questions and issues which a specialist more familiar with Japan might wish to see debated. Indeed to be successful at all we consider that the book could well raise as many questions as it sets out to answer. We realize too that readers who are expert in particular areas of the health sciences may wish to have seen that area in its Japanese context explored in greater depth. To have devoted greater attention to some topics at the expense of others would, we believe, have produced a text lacking in balance and therefore contrary to our aim, which is to provide a good introduction and general reference to the subject of health care in Japan in the 1980s.

In selecting the subject areas and topics for this book we have taken into account the need to understand that health services and their organization evolve in every country as an integral part of the political, economic, and administrative infrastructure; that they are both a reflection and an indicator of its history and present socio-cultural environment. Population size and composition, geography, and climate influence such things as the location and distribution of facilities and services. Epidemiological features change over time and must be monitored and studied so that health services best meet the needs of the population. Social and cultural factors determine individual attitudes towards health, illness, and disease and their reactions towards therapeutic and prophylactic measures. The state of a nation's economy is vitally important for the provision of health services. Many factors affect the amount of health spending in any country but economic status and policy determine the amount available from the national budget for the direct costs of providing health services. Finally, health services are not provided in a political vacuum and the allocation of resources for health care is always made within a political environment and reflects political preferences.

The book consists of nine chapters and six appendices. In the first three chapters we set the scene by offering a detailed account of the historical development of modern health services in Japan. Chapter 2 describes the major events in health and medical care in Japanese history and highlights the social and cultural factors which have affected the nature of that development. Japan experienced two centuries of self-imposed isolation from the rest of the world from the middle of the seventeenth century to the middle of the nineteenth century. From 1868, the Meiji Restoration, Japan's rulers embarked on an ambitious and carefully planned and executed programme of education and learning designed to bring the country into line with what it perceived as being the powerful and modern west.

> The Japanese determined to learn from each western country that in which it particularly excelled. For example they went to England to study the navy and the merchant marine, to Germany for the army and for medicine, to France for local government and the law and to the United States for business methods. The world was one vast schoolroom for them but they chose what and where they would learn and how they would use that knowledge to change Japan.[12]

In Chapter 3 we look at the major causes of death and disease in Japan in the 1980s, and we examine the changes that have taken place in the patterns of morbidity and mortality over the past one hundred years.

The purpose of the next three chapters is to provide an informed and critical account of the principal structural components of the health and medical services. In Chapter 4 we outline government involvement in the health services; how official policies for health are formulated and the means by which they are implemented. In Chapter 5 we outline the development of the present system of health service financing; we examine the structure and operation of the health insurance scheme and present an evaluation of its efficiency. We also touch on the appropriateness of the present system in a society undergoing rapid demographic, social, and cultural change and experiencing new demands on its rather traditional health services.

In Chapter 6 we describe the medical services delivery system and its mix of public and private hospitals and private practitioners. We look at the patterns of ownership of hospitals and clinics and note trends in the growth and distribution of such facilities. The salient features of hospital care in Japan such as length of stay, out-patient and emergency services, and some of the problems facing the hospital system will be presented.

In Chapters 7 and 8 we consider a number of key subjects; we have grouped these topics under the broad headings of the health 'industries' and the health professions. They are essential components of any health care system but in Japan perhaps more than in other countries they have evolved with certain unique characteristics and are therefore worthy of special attention.

In Chapter 7 we focus on the pharmaceutical industry in particular; after twenty years of steady growth this is now a mature industry and a major force in the economy. Like the electronics and automotive industries before it it is beginning to expand beyond Japan and to start to compete in the international market-place. Pharmaceutical products account for more than one-third of aggregate health care costs, putting Japan way ahead of most other countries. We examine therefore some of the reasons for Japan's high consumption of drugs and the relationship between the health care financing system, the pharmaceutical industry, and what has turned into an almost symbiotic relationship between the industry and the medical profession. We note too some of the new health care industries which are starting to grow.

In Chapter 8 we look at the health-care work-force; at the role of doctors, at aspects of medical education and training, and some distinctive features of medical practice in Japan. Nurses everywhere are a major part of the health work-force so we review their basic education and training and deployment within the medical care system.

In Chapter 9 we present a summary of our views on provisions for health care in Japan today and assess their suitability for the country as it enters the twenty-first century. We are all the product of our native culture, education, and environment and even as we stand back to make an assessment we carry with us the impedimenta of this background and so we offer two separate pieces in this concluding chapter, the personal findings of the two authors. We hope we thereby achieve two of the goals of this book, namely the presentation of as balanced a picture as possible and a positive contribution to harmonious Anglo-Japanese relations.

The six Appendices which provide supplemental background information are: a map of Japan, a chronology of significant historical events, exchange rate information, details of the structure of hospital ownership, and a listing of medical schools, professional organizations, and research institutions in the health sciences.

References

1 *Health and Welfare Statistics in Japan*, Tokyo, Health and Welfare Statistic Association, 1987, p. 35.
2 *Measuring Health Care 1960–1983*, Paris, OECD, 1985, p. 12.
3 J. Taylor, *Shadows of the Rising Sun: A Critical View of the Japanese Miracle*, Tokyo, C.E. Tuttle, 1983, p. 19.
4 Yasuda Mutual Life Insurance Co. Poll., *The Japan Times*, 6 November 1985.
5 *Nikkei High Tech Report*, Tokyo, Nikkei Industry Research Institute, 9 December 1985.
6 *Future Population Projections for Japan by Sex–Age, 1980–2020*, Institute of Population Problems, Tokyo, November 1981.
7 *Situation and Trends of Medical Insurance and Medical Supply in Japan*, Tokyo, National Federation of Health Insurance Societies, 1985.
8 *Japan in the Year 2000: Preparing Japan for the Age of Internationalisation, the Aging Society and Maturity*, Long-Term Outlook Committee, Economic Council, Economic Planning Agency, Japan Times Ltd, 1983, pp. 14–15.
9 E.O. Reischauer, *Japan: Past and Present*, New York, Alfred A. Knopf, 1946.
10 B. Abel-Smith, *Value for Money in the Health Services*, London, Heinemann Educational Books, 1976, Preface.
11 M.E. Roemer, *Health Care Systems in World Perspective*, Ann Arbor, Mich., Health Administration Press, 1976, p. 3.
12 E.O. Reischauer, *Japan: The Story of a Nation*, Tokyo, C.E. Tuttle, 1976, p. 135. (First published as *Japan: Past and Present*, New York, Alfred A. Knopf, 1946.)

Chapter two

The history of medical care in Japan

Until the end of the Tokugawa Shogunate in 1868 Chinese medicine – kanpo – was the type of systematized medical care practised in Japan. Although it comprised the same techniques as those used in mainland China – acupuncture, moxibustion, finger pressure therapy, massage, and herbal medicines – the brand of Chinese medicine offered in Japan was not a mere copy of the original because it had, in the course of time, been modified and improved upon and generally made more compatible with Japanese conditions. Some knowledge of the essence of Chinese medicine will contribute to an understanding of why its practice fell out of favour; there were some important developments in medical care in Japan prior to the Meiji Restoration which caused Japanese physicians to reconsider the whole system of medical care in the country and to be so receptive to a second foreign model of medical and health care.

History of Chinese medicine in China[1,2]

The origins of Chinese medicine are thought to date back to legendary times earlier than 2260 BC. It is said that the first Emperor Hu Hsi, the peak of whose reign was approximately 2910 BC, advocated a primitive doctrine of the Yin and the Yang, which was to become the philosophical basis of Chinese thought including medical theories.

The second Emperor and 'Divine Peasant' Shen Nong, whose reign reached its pinnacle in 2780 BC, is said to have compiled *Shen Nong's Herbal* or *The Herbal* (Shen Nong Ben Cao Jing), the earliest materia medica in which 365 kinds of drugs were listed and divided into three classes: superior, medium (common), and inferior. Later studies established that this book was a product of the first century BC.

Huang-di's Internal Classic or *Canon of Medicine* (Huang-di Nei Jing) is the oldest and greatest classic work extant in China, with its authorship attributed to the third Emperor Huang-di (2698–2589 BC). The book was written in the form of questions and answers or dialogues between the Emperor and six famous physicians and consists of two parts: 'Plain Questions' (Su Wen) and 'Miraculous Pivot' known as 'Canon of Acupuncture' (Ling Shu). Again further research suggests that the work was a product of various unknown authors in the Warring States period (475–221 BC). The theories and therapies of this classical work were mainly developed in the region to the north of the Yellow River (Huang Ho) and were grounded in metaphysical, abstract, and idealistic philosophy, encompassing theories on the unification of nature and human beings, the Yin and the Yang, the five natural elements and so on. Acupuncture and moxibustion were the principal therapies advocated in this school of medicine.

Another school of thought developed from the work and teachings of Zhang Zhong Jing (AD 150?–219?), one of the most influential physicians in the history of Chinese medicine. He collected information on symptoms and the outcome of therapies such as herbal preparations which were in widespread use along the Yangtze River and in areas to the south of it. He advocated methods of analysing and differentiating pathological conditions in accordance with the six channels and the eight principal syndromes. His treatise was a pioneering work on the principles of treating diseases according to the differentiation of signs and symptoms. He wrote several other books of which the most important was *Treatise on Fevers and Miscellaneous Diseases* (Shang Han Za Bing Lun). Written at the beginning of the third century AD it dealt extensively with the diagnosis and treatment of fevers and other common diseases; it extended over sixteen volumes and was entitled *Treatise on Febrile Diseases* (Shang Han Lun). The practice of mainstream, traditional Chinese medicine was based therefore on the two aforementioned classical works – *Huang-di's Internal Classic* or *Canon of Medicine* (Huang-di Nei Jing) and the *Treatise on Febrile Diseases* (Shang Han Lun) – and consisted consequently of two principal schools of thought and practice. Theory was largely drawn from the former work and practice from the latter.

Although there were some slight modifications, developments, and new interpretations to these basic theories there were no great changes in the practice of Chinese medicine until the periods of the Chin (AD 1115–1234) and the Yuan (AD 1234–1368) dynasties when attempts were made to unify the traditional therapies of acupuncture and moxibustion with herbal therapy. In the Chin period the School of Cathartic, advocating offensive and cooling therapy, was formed. Then in the Yuan period, as a compromise, a school advocating passive or defensive and warming therapy, the so-called School of Nourishing, was formed. This school was called the Li-Zhu School from the names of its two founders. The school was influential through the Ming (AD 1368–1644) and Ching (AD 1662–1911) dynasties up until the present time. It was this school that was introduced into Japan in the sixteenth century and opened up a new era for Chinese medicine in Japan.

Introduction of Chinese medicine in Japan[3,4]

In ancient times the Japanese developed their own primitive medical beliefs and practices which included anatomical dissections and autopsies. However after Buddhism arrived in the country no anatomical dissections were performed until the middle of the eighteenth century. According to Chinese records the ancient Japanese were a healthy people who enjoyed long lives and were aware of the importance of cleanliness in preventing the spread of disease. The development of purification rituals is said to be derived from this.

From earliest times Japan was in contact with her mainland neighbours Korea and China, which were more advanced and civilized in all areas. Until the sixth century knowledge about Chinese medicine came to Japan largely through Koreans and in the middle of the sixth century the reception of a Korean mission at the Japanese court marked the first official entry of Buddhism and other components of Chinese culture and civilization into Japan. Direct communication between China and Japan grew from this time and Buddhist medico-priests were among the many travellers from the mainland, especially during the periods of the Sui (AD 589–617) and Tang (AD 618–959) dynasties when China enjoyed remarkable prosperity and prestige. Japan's political and intellectual leaders were eager to adopt and copy all things Chinese; Japan's citizens were perhaps less happy that contact with China also brought with it the introduction of new diseases, e.g. measles. Chinese medicine at the time was closely connected with Buddhism: charity institutions including hospitals were established in the precincts of Buddhist temples and medico-priests and nurse-priests were produced in great numbers.

The Medical Law included in the Taiho Codes of 701 recommended nationalization of health services under the control of a Director of Medical and Pharmaceutical Affairs of the Ministry of the Imperial Household and that medical officers be sent to provincial capitals. The code also specified a system of medical education and the establishment of schools in both national and provincial capitals. Training for medical officers was to last for seven years for internal medicine, five years for paediatrics and surgery, seven years for acupuncture, three years for massage, and three years for magical or religious therapies. Female physicians and nurses were also to be trained. A system to monitor the outbreak and spread of epidemics was also inaugurated and provisions also specified the duties of individuals in relation to the care of relatives aged 80 or over or who were seriously ill.

In its early days in Japan Chinese medicine was monopolized by the Imperial family and the noble classes. But treatment gradually spread among the people who none the less continued to rely for some time on native practices such as faith-healing. With some adaptations and Japanese innovations Chinese medicine was to be the principal form of systematized medical care in the country until the beginning of the Tokugawa or Edo period (1600–1868). During the Kamakura period (1185–1336) the samurai gained power from the aristocracy and Buddhism was at the peak of its influence; at this time private medical practice expanded and Buddhist charity medical activities were widespread. The country was beset by frequent civil wars from the Namboku period (1336–92) right through to the Muromachi period (1392–1573) and medical practice saw considerable improvements in the areas of practical surgery for the treatment of injury and the introduction of specialized practice for ophthalmology, obstetrics–gynaecology, and paediatrics.

The development of Chinese medicine in Japan[4]

By 1868 when the Meiji government decreed the adoption of western medicine, the foundations for this programme of modernization of the Japanese medical care system had already been laid. First, the practice of Chinese medicine had been subject to innovations and had changed its fundamental nature under the influence of new ideas and criticism from its more creative proponents and leading thinkers. Second, Spanish and Portugese missionary medicine, and later Dutch medicine practised by the medical officers in the Dutch enclave on Dejima Island in Nagasaki Harbour, had demonstrated the effectiveness of other approaches in the diagnosis and treatment of disease and the treatment of injury. Many physicians who practised Chinese medicine, and particularly those who adhered to the positivist Classicist school, were receptive to embracing aspects of 'rampo' or western medicine. We will examine first the changes which had taken place in the practice of Chinese medicine in Japan and the development of the Classicist School of Medicine.

For most of the Edo era (1600–1868) the dominant school of Chinese medicine was the Latter Day School of Medicine (Koseiho or Goseiho). The founder of this school was Sanki Tashiro (1465–1537), who spent more than ten years in China during the Ming Dynasty (1368–1644). His studies in China focused on a type of medicine which had been developed in the Jin (1125–1234) and Yuan (1279–1368) dynasties, particularly the medicine of the Li-Zhu school, named after its two founders. It was Tashiro's most prominent follower, Dosan Manase (1507–95), who further developed and enhanced the Yin-Yuan medicine of the Li-Zhu school in Japan. This Latter Day School of Medicine departed from Buddhist principles and became based in Confucianism, which took over as the fundamental ideology of the Tokugawa Shogunates. This school was particularly important for the furtherance of a Japanese medicine which was relatively independent and no longer a mere imitation of its Chinese original. But practitioners of this school soon became entrenched in their views and the school as a whole tended towards impractical idealism. Moreover all the physicians for the Shogunate were selected from the followers of this school and it gradually became troubled by corrupt practices.

Criticism of the Latter Day School of Medicine led to the development of the so-called Classicist School (Koiho), the emergence of which hailed the complete Japanicization of traditional Chinese medicine in the country. The Classicist school esteemed the positivist approach of the Classical Shang Han Lun and took as its motto 'Return to the Classical Shang Han Lun'. The school was radically reformative and produced many prominent physicians who invented new techniques and made several important medical discoveries. Many of its practitioners subsequently combined the techniques of Japanese medicine with Dutch medicine and thus were instrumental in paving the way for the successful introduction of western medical practice after the Meiji Restoration.

Two influential predecessors to this school were Joun Saka (birth and death dates unknown) and Tokumoto Nagata (1513(?)–1630). The former was born to a famous family of physicians, studied in China during the Ming dynasty in the early 1490s, and introduced the medical theory of Shang Han Lun to Japan. Nagata achieved considerable fame in the country, because of his excellent care and treatment, especially his prescription of drugs; a modest individual who did not seek personal wealth or fame, he was renowned for his habit of travelling on the back of a cow to treat his patients. He was bitterly critical of many of his fellow physicians who often seemed more concerned about fame and fortune than about treating the sick. He cared for members of the Tokugawa Shogunate and is credited with saving the life of the Shogun, refusing all gifts and payments for his services other than his normal fee of 18 mon (the currency of the times).

The principal founders of the Classicist School are held to be Kozan Goto (1655–1733) and his chief pupil Shutoku Kagawa (1683–1755), who emphasized the importance of observation and experiment and established the positivist foundation of medical practice. Goto dissected animals in order to carry out thorough studies of anatomy at a time when human dissection was prohibited. Kagawa rejected all abstract concepts relating to the body such as the doctrine of the Yin and Yang and that of the five elements and was highly critical of all the medical classics of the day including the Shang Han Lun. He was a great believer and proponent of therapeutic bathing, stipulating quite detailed recommendations on the correct and most efficacious bathing practice. Among their distinguished pupils were Todo Yoshimasu (1702–73), who was famous for his innovative clinical studies, and Toyo Yamawaki (1705–62), who was the first Japanese to carry out a human dissection on the body of a dead criminal at Rokkaku prison in 1754. He was deeply impressed by the accuracy of the anatomical charts in a Dutch version of an anatomy textbook by Johanan Vesling (a German-born professor at the University of Padua) when he compared the charts with his own findings. He published his account of the dissection some five years later, including anatomical illustrations. Those who were influenced by Yamawaki's teachings were to play an important role in the later introduction of western medicine. The Classicist School produced a number of prominent physicians worthy of mention because of their original discoveries or inventions and their contribution to the progress of Japanese medical care. Gen'etsu Kagawa (1700–77) published a treatise entitled *Sanron* (The Principles of Obstetrics) in 1766 in which he correctly described the normal inverted position of the foetus in the uterus and other techniques or principles of obstetric practice. Soteki Fuseya (1747–1811) carried out various experiments to establish how the kidneys work and the urinogenous process; he disclosed his findings in 1805. Seishu Hanaoka (1760–1835) performed an operation on a breast cancer in 1805 successfully using an anaesthetic preparation of his own invention. He worked for some twenty years perfecting this compound of six crude drugs from the traditional Chinese medicine pharmacopoeia and went on to use the 'mafutsusan' in numerous surgical procedures in the treatment of malignant tumours, haemorrhoids, gangrene, anal prolapse, and so on. All this successful research and experiment was carried out by the Japanese, often earlier than similar work by their western contemporaries and without the benefit of information about the developments taking place in the western world at the time.

The roots of western medicine in Japan[4]

The second thread which paved the way for the establishment of modern western medical practice in Japan was the direct influence of European and Christian missionary medicine. It was in 1542 or 1543 when some Portugese mariners heading for Macao were driven ashore on an island called Tanegashima off the southern tip of Kyushu that the Japanese saw their first European and the first contact between Japan and the west was made. The arrival of the Portugese was an event which would have massive and far-reaching repercussions for the Japanese. First and obviously came trade with the outside world; a more significant phenomenon was the introduction of firearms whose use spread rapidly through the country and greatly altered the nature of warfare and the outcome of the seemingly endless feuds between rival lords. Next were the educational, medical, and other activities of the Portugese and Spanish missionaries who soon started to arrive in Japan; Francis Xavier the distinguished Jesuit was one of the early missionaries.

In 1557 the first western-style hospital was built at what is now Oita, Kyushu by the Portugese missionary physician Luis de Almeida (1525–84) who arrived in Japan in 1555. A skilled and knowledgeable surgeon, he soon started to train his Japanese helpers, usually making them responsible for internal medicine. The hospital started from the pharmacy which he had established using medicines shipped in from Macao. In its heyday the hospital was treating more than one hundred in-patients and had a staff of four European and four Japanese doctors. Similar missionary facilities were soon built in different parts of the country and quickly became very popular with the Japanese people. Although the missionary doctors were not always as skilled or as up-to-date as their colleagues back in Europe they undoubtedly provided better and more effective treatment than that offered by the practitioners of traditional Chinese medicine. The missionaries moreover went out of their way to help the poorer classes, who suffered particularly fiercely from the physical impact of civil wars and unrest. They were attracted by both the quality of the medical care given and the humanitarian spirit which informed it.

The majority of the early missionaries were Jesuits but they were soon prohibited from practising medicine by holy orders which arrived in Japan in 1560. In 1587 the Shogun Hideyoshi issued a decree ordering all Christians to leave Japan and missionary medical activities started to fall off. But it was not until 1639 and the adoption of the strict isolationist policy by the Tokugawa Shogunate that missionary hospitals finally became extinct. However western medicine ('nanban' or southern medicine) introduced by these missionaries did manage to survive, particularly surgical techniques which were of undoubted usefulness and value to the Japanese. It was this 'nanban' combined with Dutch medicine which provided the foundation for modern western medicine.

Introduction and dissemination of Dutch medicine[4,5]

By the turn of the sixteenth century Spain and Portugal were losing their hegemony over the seven seas to the growing power of Holland and Britain. At this time too Japan was beginning its persecution of the Spanish and Portugese missionaries, who were considered a dangerous threat and rival to the established Buddhist religion and were held to pose a political threat to the Shogunate by harbouring possible territorial ambitions. After the decree banning Christian missionaries in 1587 little was done actively to remove them from the country but in 1614 Shogun Ieyasu reinstated executions of missionaries and native converts. The persecution of Christians came to a head in 1637 and 1638, when Christian peasants in Shimabara in Kyushu rebelled in desperation over economic and religious persecution. The brutal suppression of the rebellion marked the end of Christianity as a form of religion in Japan. In 1636 the Japanese were prohibited from going overseas and foreigners were forbidden from entering the country. With the prohibition on the building of ocean-going vessels in 1639 Japan's isolationist policy was complete. For the sake of profit and in order to maintain some contact with the outside world the Tokugawa Shogunate allowed the Dutch and the Chinese to carry on trade with Japan under severely restricted conditions. All foreigners were confined to Dejima, an artificial island in Nagasaki harbour. After the Japanese had cut themselves off so comprehensively from the rest of the world it was through one channel only, the Dutch Trading House on Dejima, that limited information and knowledge about European science including medicine trickled back into Japan.

The Dutch government made it a rule to send a medical officer (Opperchirurgijn) to Dejima in order to care for members of the Dutch trading house and their families. Each medical officer's assignment lasted on average two to three years. From 1641 when the first medical officer arrived in Dejima to 1858 when the last one left the country more than one hundred medical officers served the Dejima community. These medical officers were also a valuable source of information on European science in general as well as on European medical practice; their knowledge and teaching were disseminated by their Japanese interpreters, many of whom in fact became physicians by taking advantage of their knowledge of Dutch and their privilege of working with the Dutch doctors. Learning Dutch was initially limited to the spoken language and Japanese interpreters were not allowed to study the written language; this prohibition was repealed in 1739 by the Eighth Shogun Yoshimitsu and from that time Nagasaki and specifically Dejima and the interpreters' houses became centres of Dutch studies which soon expanded to encompass western learning in general; medicine was one field of study which grew in importance. Students at this time were selected by feudal lords from all over Japan.

The Dutch government seemed to select and send capable physicians to Dejima as a matter of diplomatic policy. There were therefore a number of prominent physicians in the settlement who fulfilled a dual role; they contributed to the development of Japanese medicine and furthered the cause of Japanese studies back in Europe. Among the physicians sent to Dejima can be counted several famous and influential non-Dutch Europeans – Germans and Swedes who entered Japan classified as Dutch and including Casper Schambruger, who stayed in Japan from 1649 to 1651 and taught several Japanese interpreters Dutch medicine, primarily surgery which became known as the Casper school of surgery. He also influenced developments in astronomy and surveying. Willem ten Rhyne (1647–1700), who was invited to treat the fourth Shogun Iyetsuna of the Tokugawa family, stayed in Japan from 1675 to 1676 and later introduced things Japanese, including traditional Chinese medicine, to Europe. Englebert Kaempfer (1651–1716), a German physician and historian, was in Japan from 1690 to 1692; he taught Dutch medicine, did research into Japanese culture and natural history, and became one of Europe's most distinguished Japanese scholars. Karl Peter Thunberg (1743–1828), who lived in Japan from 1775 to 1776, was a Swede and a student of the renowned Swedish botanist Carl Linnaeus. Thunberg came to Japan with the intention of carrying out comprehensive studies of all aspects of Japanese life and especially traditional medicine, plants, and animals. His influence on the development of Dutch or western studies in Japan was so strong that he has been acknowledged as an early founder of western medicine in the country.

One of the most influential among all the medical officers of the Dutch Trading House was Phillip Franz von Siebold (1796–1866), a German who lived in Japan twice, during 1823–9 and 1859–61. His enthusiasm, breadth of knowledge, and fine character greatly moved his Japanese students and so impressed the local feudal governor that he was granted exceptional privileges, being allowed for example to teach and practise medicine outside the Dejima. He amassed an extensive collection of Japanese artefacts, accepting them as payment from his Japanese patients, including objects which were normally prohibited for export. When he left Japan for Europe his ship was wrecked and his collection of treasures discovered. As a consequence he was deported and his thirty-two Japanese followers who had helped him find his collection were arrested and punished. Under the new Dutch-Japanese Treaty of Commerce in 1858 he returned to Japan with his son and became a diplomatic adviser to the Shogunate. He devoted himself to his Japanese studies again and was instrumental in disseminating information about Japan in Europe. Many of his Japanese students who came from various parts of the country went on to become leaders and pioneers of western medicine and science in the country.

Another memorable medical officer was Otto Mohnicke (1814–87), who lived in Japan from 1848 to 1850 and introduced Jenner's anti-smallpox vaccine into the country. The introduction of the smallpox vaccine and the use of the stethoscope were critical factors in the acceptance of western medical knowledge in the country and its gradual subjugation of traditional Chinese medicine. An anti-smallpox vaccination centre established at Otamagaike in Edo in 1858 with funds donated by eighty-two physicians of the Dutch school was taken over by the Shogunate as the western medical centre in 1860. This facility was the forerunner of the Medical Faculty of the University of Tokyo which subsequently became the pre-eminent medical school for teaching western medicine in Japan.

A notable event in the history of the introduction of Dutch or western medicine in Japan was the publication of the Japanese translation of the Dutch version of a German anatomy textbook written by Johann Adam Kulmus (1689–1745) in 1722. This text was widely read in Europe at the time and besides the Dutch version there were Latin and French texts. The Japanese title was *Kaitai Shinsho* (The New Book on Human Anatomy). The Japanese translation was done by Genpaku Sugita and other scholars of the School of Dutch Studies (called Rangaku). In 1771 Sugita and his friend Ryotaku Maeno, a scholar of Dutch medicine, observed the dissection of the body of a woman criminal who had been executed. Each of them had a copy of Kulmus' textbook and were impressed by the accuracy of the descriptions in the work, so much so that they decided to embark on a Japanese translation. As their knowledge of Dutch was limited it took them three years of hard work to complete the project. After the publication of 'Kaitai Shinsho' in 1774 more than 1,500 western medical books, the majority of Dutch provenance, were translated into Japanese and formed the basis of Japanese explorations in western medical science. The success of western medicine in Japan in these early days can therefore be attributed to the work of such individual enthusiastic scholars as these.

The development and dissemination of Dutch medicine did not always progress smoothly. Physicians of the authorized dominant school of Chinese medicine, many of whom held positions as official physicians to the Shogun, were apprehensive about the incursion of Dutch medicine and jealous of its obvious successes. They were able to influence the Shogunate sufficiently to cause the official suppression of Dutch medicine from 1839 to 1854. However, as we have seen, Japan's isolation from the rest of the world was soon to come to an end and her by-now native system of medical care was but one aspect of her culture which was destined to be comprehensively reformed. In the 250 years of the Tokugawa Shogunate traditional Chinese medicine in Japan had grown into a scientific entity which was much broader than its original Chinese model and, as we have seen, it was also changing as a result of the acquisition of new knowledge, albeit limited and arriving sporadically, from the western world. Provision of medical care to the greater part of the country's population had not advanced a great deal and was for the most part poor indeed. There were no hospitals for the care of the sick and most medical practitioners, no matter what brand of medicine they practised, generally confined their endeavours to the ruling or noble classes.

The by-now declining influence of traditional Chinese medicine 'kampo' was dealt a decisive blow by a number of factors and the way thus prepared for the formal adoption of the German system of medical care, which was to prove influential until 1945. First was the evident success of Jennerian vaccine in the treatment of smallpox; second, western drugs were manifestly more successful in the treatment of some diseases than kampo's concoctions; third, physicians of the Dutch school were appointed to supervise the care and treatment of the thirteenth Shogun Iesada Tokugawa when he was terminally ill; finally in formally adopting western-style military training officialdom acknowledged the superiority of a body of knowledge that was not Japanese.

In 1857 the Shogunate appointed a Dutch naval-surgeon Pompe van Meerdervoort (1829–1908) as medical instructor at the government naval school in Nagasaki. For five years he taught a comprehensive curriculum in western medicine ranging from basic science, human anatomy, and dissection through to practical clinical training to a body of students who had been chosen by feudal lords from all over the country. Meerdervoort was succeeded by A.F. Bauduin and C.G. van Mansvelt successively, also Dutch physicians. This school was the forerunner of the medical school of Nagasaki University and its graduates became prominent in medical circles in the new era in Japan. If it can be said that Siebold sowed the seeds of western medicine in Japan then Meerdervoort can justifiably be credited with having ensured the right conditions for it to germinate in Japanese soil.

Health, illness, and health care in the Shogun era[6]

In the previous section we described prominent individuals and practitioners who influenced trends and developments in Japanese medical care rather than the doctors and therapists who served the general public. In feudal times anyone could practise as a physician simply by proclaiming himself to be one; no particular qualifications or education were necessary. Physicians were roughly divided into two groups: those employed as court retainers by the feudal lords, and private practitioners including traditional healers who lived and worked among the population at large. The level of medical knowledge and technical skill varied enormously, as might be expected. There were medical practitioners whose knowledge was limited to what they had read in a couple of textbooks or picked up from a friend or relative; on the other hand many were highly skilled, well educated and informed, actively pursued new knowledge, and were innovators. For the majority of the general public the traditional Chinese practitioner was the usual source of help in times of illness. Individual patients usually paid the doctor twice a year: in the middle of the summer and at the end of the year, and payment was considered to be for the drugs dispensed rather than for any treatment or advice given. There is only a limited amount of information about the health status of the population at that time. It is supposed that the average diet was lacking in protein. Epidemics of smallpox and influenza are known to be the principal threats to the overall health of the population.

Modern Japan 1868–1945[7-13]

Japanese society has undergone revolutionary change twice in modern times: the Meiji Restoration in 1868 and the country's defeat in 1945 each ushered in times of substantial social, political, and economic change. In the period 1868 to 1945 when Japan developed into a modern capitalist industrial society, several distinct phases can be distinguished in which the prevailing social and political conditions influenced specific developments or introduced changes in the health care services. The stages can be distinguished as follows:

1 1868–90: a period of rapid modernization; the adoption and absorption of German medicine; spread of acute epidemics and lack of quarantine regulations at the main ports of entry.
2 1890–1930: industrial revolution and economic depression; Sino-Japanese, Russo-Japanese wars; social problems and unrest; labour and socialist movements gain momentum. Independence of Japanese medicine. The so-called 'golden' years for Japanese physicians. Movement for the socialization of medical care, charity medical care. Health insurance (for employees) law.
3 1930–40: rise of militarism. Defeat in Second World War. National Health Insurance Law and expansion of health insurance coverage; wartime health care system.

1868–90: The Meiji Restoration and Japan's modernization[5,14–17]

We have seen that despite the official seclusion policy Japan was not entirely cut off from the outside world during the Tokugawa Shogunate. In medicine the work and teaching of the Dutch physicians attached to the enclave on Dejima helped to introduce western medical ideas and practice into the country.

By the middle of the nineteenth century the foundations of Japan's feudalistic society were being eroded by internal and external pressures. There was a revival of emperor-centred nationalism supported by the court nobility in Kyoto. The authority of the Shogunate was also threatened by the growth of a merchant capitalist class in the cities and towns and simmering unrest among the urban poor and the rural peasants. However a decisive role in the eventual overthrow of the Shogunate was to be played by the low-ranking, frustrated, and radical samurai of the 'outer feudal clans', together with pressure from western powers demanding the opening up of the country for trade and commerce.

In 1853 an American squadron of four 'Black ships' under Commodore Matthew C. Perry (1794–1858) and a Russian expedition of four vessels led by Admiral Evfimii Vasilievich Putyatin (1803–83) appeared in Japanese waters and demanded that Japan commence trade with their countries. These demands were initially refused despite the assertions of the foreigners that they would return with stronger forces the following year. The Americans were particularly keen to establish 'bases' in Japan as it lay on the route to China with whom it was seriously developing trade; Japan was important for the requisition of supplies for the merchant marine. The ultimatum delivered by both commanders threw the Shogunate into a state of turmoil with the two main opposing factions arguing either for or against agreement to the demands of the foreigners. By the time that Perry returned to Japan with seven ships in February 1854 the realists had gained the upper hand and a treaty was signed in Yokohama on 31 March 1854. The terms of the treaty opened up two ports – Shimoda and Hakodate – to American ships for supplies and trade. Shipwrecked seamen were to be protected and an American Consul was to be stationed in Shimoda. The British concluded a treaty in October of the same year, opening up Nagasaki and Hakodate to British vessels for supplies. The Russians concluded a treaty in February 1855 which included agreement on the northern borders and opened up three ports – Nagasaki, Shimoda, and Hakodate – to Russian vessels.

Diplomatic demands from the USA, Russia, Britain, and other nations escalated thereafter and various treaties eventually allowed foreigners into Edo (Tokyo), exempted them from the Japanese courts of law, and allowed them greatly reduced import taxes. The treaties were called 'the unequal treaties' and their revision was a major aim of Japanese foreign policy until the end of the nineteenth century.

The decade from 1858 was a time of tension, confusion, and civil wars as the opposing factions sought to gain the upper hand. Finally an alliance of feudatories from western Japan led by young samurai and supported by the Kyoto nobles and Osaka merchant families overthrew the Shogunate and supreme power was restored to the Emperor. This was the Meiji Restoration. Before the Restoration foreigners from several countries had been employed by both sides of the warring factions; Britain favoured the unification of Japan under the Emperor and had supported the anti-Tokugawa clans – the Choshu and the Satsuma – who were to produce the dominant leaders in early Meiji times. Dr Willis of the British legation in Yokohama treated injured soldiers of the anti-Shogunate clans and impressed their leaders with the excellence of his treatment and the effectiveness of his medicine. France on the other hand had sympathies for the Shogunate and provided assistance with training and advice on military matters to the Shogun's armies.

After the Meiji Restoration the Japanese government engaged increasing numbers of western specialists in many fields, including medicine, to help the country to modernize and catch up with the technologically advanced nations of the west. While the events of the time were indeed revolutionary for Japan, Japan's revolution was perhaps not a true one and the word 'restoration' succinctly suggests both the limitations of the revolution and its subtle distinctions from the social revolutions which had preceded it in Europe, for example the bourgeois revolution in France. It was in many respects an imperfect revolution right from the start, as the majority of the population was not directly involved in it – the feudal regime was not overthrown by a rising bourgeoisie. It heralded Japan's rather late embarkation on the voyage of modernization and industrialization, one guided moreover by fear of further encroachment by foreign powers, not necessarily rooted in a desire for a modern society *per se*. The modernization programme was government inspired and led 'top-down', and informed by the official slogan of 'a rich country and a strong army'. It was against this social and political background that Japan's modern health care began.

Adoption of western medicine – German medicine as a model[7,18]

In accordance with the Imperial Covenant of March 1868 and the precept 'knowledge shall be sought for [sic] all over the world and thus shall be strengthened the foundation of the imperial policy', the newly born government proclaimed permission for the practice of western medicine in March. This implied the active adoption of western medicine and the renunciation of Chinese medicine which had been officially acknowledged by the Tokugawa Shogunate. Pragmatic militaristic requirements informed this decision. The new government leaders had observed and been impressed by the superiority and greater effectiveness of western medicine in dealing with the war-wounded during the civil wars. Masujiro Ohmura, a founder of the modern Japanese army, was also a physician and had some experience of Dutch medicine.

The government next appointed two physicians who had studied Dutch medicine in Nagasaki, Jun Iwasa and Chian Sagara, to draft and recommend a programme to reform medical care and medical education. They decided on the adoption of German medicine and thus paved the way for drastic change in Japanese medical care. In his memoirs Chian Sagara noted seven reasons for recommending the adoption of German medicine; the sixth and seventh reasons were as follows:

> Six. . . . Japan could not afford to follow the French elegance because of Japan's economic status.
>
> Seven. . . . In those days the Netherlands was politically weak and many of the Dutch medical books were in any case translations of German and French books; the British despised the Japanese; the United States was such a young country that medicine had not developed much, whereas Germany resembled Japan in polity or political regime and was new to Asia. Therefore it seemed appropriate that German medicine be chosen.
>
> (Japan Ministry of Health and Welfare, 1925)

Besides these obviously political reasons German medicine was realistically judged to be the most advanced in Europe; the German language was similar to Dutch with which many of Japan's enlightened physicians were already familiar and thus the switch to German could be relatively uncomplicated. Even British medicine, which had been quite influential thanks to the work of Dr Willis, was deserted for the reasons given above.

In February 1870 the Japanese drew up a contract to employ two Prussian medical instructors. The Franco-Prussian War delayed their arrival somewhat, causing some frustration among the government and students alike as they were desperately anxious to get on with the modernization of Japanese medicine as speedily as possible. The two instructors, Benjamin Carl Leopold Müller (1824–93), Surgeon First Lieutenant, and Theodor Eduard Hoffmann (1837–?), Second Assistant Surgeon, arrived in 1871 and began to teach at the forerunner of the Medical School at Tokyo University.

The two instructors were empowered with full authority to establish the new medical education system at Tokyo University. They were granted exceptional privileges and were responsible to nobody but the Minister of Education in their teachings and decisions. Some idea of their elevated position can be judged from the fact that their monthly salary of 600 yen exceeded that paid to senior cabinet ministers at the time. The programme of medical education which they developed was closely modelled on the German army medical education provided at the Friedrich Wilhelm Institute and was stricter and more dogmatic than the system of medical education offered in German universities. The medical course at Tokyo University comprised two years preparatory course and five years of regular medical education. Müller lectured in surgery and taught anatomy and pathology. These two left Japan at the end of their two-year contract and they were replaced by other German instructors. By now the abler Japanese students were being sent to Germany to study. In the mean time the administrative and legal foundations of the country's modern medical care system were being formed. In 1872 the Medical Section was established in the Ministry of Education and its status raised to that of Medical Bureau the following year, with Chian Sagara as the first Director. The Medical Law, the first fundamental statute in modern Japan, was prepared by the Ministry of Education and enacted in 1874. The main contents and aims were

1 organization of the health administrative structure under the control of the Ministry of Education,
2 establishment of the medical education system modelled on western medicine,
3 inauguration of a licensing system for medical practitioners,

4 foundation of a modern drug control administration system and the system of separation of prescription of drugs by medical practitioners from dispensary at pharmacies.

Tokyo University centred modernization of medical education[19]

Among the administrative reforms undertaken at the time were the abolition of the feudal fief system and the introduction of the prefectural system of local government in 1871; in 1872 conscription was adopted and the Education Law enacted; in 1873 the modern land tax system was introduced.

Tokyo University now became the national centre for the modernization of Japan through the educational system. The Education Law introduced the regional university system, which divided the country into five regions for the purposes of education administration. The forerunner of Tokyo University School of Medicine was the First University Regional Medical School. Regions Two and Three had no school. Osaka and Nagasaki Medical Schools were set up for Regions Four and Five but were abolished in 1872 and 1874 respectively. Thus by 1874 the forerunner of the Tokyo University School of Medicine was the only medical school under direct government control through the Ministry of Education. In 1877 the Medical School and the Tokyo Kaisei School (the centre for law, liberal arts, and the sciences) were merged to become the Tokyo University.

While these developments were taking place in the nation's capital there were also some relatively strong local autonomous efforts to establish medical education and care. In 1871 when the fiefs were abolished, 98 out of the 272 clans or feudatories in the country had introduced some form of medical education system. Thirty or so had introduced Dutch and other varieties of Western medicine and hired foreign instructors and physicians. The number of public and private medical schools grew rapidly and by 1879 there were 20 public and 25 private institutions with more than 3,000 students. Several hundred Japanese and a handful of foreigners were employed as instructors; local medical schools were however keen to employ graduates of Tokyo University Medical School and consequently offered generous salaries and benefits as incentives to lure them to the provinces.

Further official steps were taken to achieve institutional supremacy of Tokyo University and of particular importance was the examination exemption system which was introduced to consolidate the system of medical licensure. From 1876 licence to practise was granted only to those trained in western medical science. This of course excluded the kanpo practitioners who were still the majority. They formed an association to press for inclusion in the new system but against a background of officially endorsed modernism they were unsuccessful and by the end of the century were a spent force in mainstream health care. In 1879 examination exemption was granted for graduates of various European universities and for those who had graduated from national university medical schools in Japan, only Tokyo University at the time. In 1882 the examination exemption was expanded to include those graduates of medical schools which had at least three graduates of the university medical school on the teaching staff; in effect only Tokyo University graduates qualified. In 1883 the medical practitioners' examination exemption applied only to graduates of the national and public university medical schools and as a result the number of private medical schools went into decline. By 1884 there were thirty public medical schools and only two private medical schools remained – Saisei Gakusha and the Seikai Koshuujo. The latter was to become the Jikei Medical College in Tokyo. These two private schools were remarkable institutions. Saisei Gakusha was founded in 1876 by Tai Hasegawa, a retired medical professor, administrator, and politician, as a preparatory school for the medical practitioners' examinations. By the time of its closure in 1902 a total of 15,000 students out of an enrolment of 21,000 had passed the necessary examinations and qualified as medical practitioners; an unusually large proportion of the graduates of this school went on to become highly influential members in local medical association activities. The Seikai Koshuujo was established by Kanehiro Takagi who had received his medical education in England and the curriculum at his school was therefore closer to the British model than to the prevailing German one.

The early years of the Meiji regime saw sharp inflation because of colossal military expenditure and heavy spending on educational and other developmental programmes. Management of medical schools soon became a financial burden to the newly established prefectural governments and there was a decline in their numbers from thirty in 1884 to twenty-six in 1886 and eighteen in 1887. Finally a government ordinance of 1887 banned the subsidy of prefectural medical schools from prefectural taxes. Only three financially sound schools survived, namely Aichi (the present Nagoya University School of Medicine), Kyoto (now Kyoto Municipal Medical College), and Osaka (the present Osaka University School of Medicine).

In 1886 the Imperial University Ordinance designated Tokyo University as Japan's sole Imperial University. Thus was established the pyramidal structure of medical education in Japan, with Tokyo Imperial University School of Medicine at the top followed by the regional national medical schools, the three above-mentioned surviving prefectural medical schools, and finally the remaining private medical schools. This structure continued to prevail until the present day.

Foundation of hospitals[20,21]

Prior to the Meiji Restoration the only institutions for the care and treatment of sick people had been the Christian missionary hospitals set up from the middle of the sixteenth century through to the early seventeenth century, and the hospital built in Nagasaki towards the end of the Edo era on the advice of Pompe van Meerdervoort.

In 1868 military hospitals were built in Kyoto, Osaka, and Yokohama. Later on as part of the modernization policy feudal lords and subsequently the prefectural governments built public hospitals, most of them attached to medical schools. As we can see in Table 2.1, in the early Meiji period the public hospitals outnumbered the private facilities. However after 1887 and the Ordinance banning support for prefectural medical schools from prefectural taxes, many prefectural hospitals were closed. The number of private hospitals then started to outgrow the number of public hospitals.

The public hospitals were initially set up, like their European counterparts, to provide treatment for the poor. However the high calibre of the medical staff and superior facilities increasingly attracted middle- and upper-class patients. Just as the system of education and training was modelled on the German so too the hospitals shared some of the characteristics of their models. Outpatient departments were important because they provided research and training material for the staff. There was often little co-operation between clinical departments. Medical care for the poorer classes was left in the hands of the kanpo practitioners and a growing number of physician-owned clinics; it was thus that Japan's private-sector-dominated pattern of medical care delivery was established.

The opening up of the ports and the arrival of large numbers of foreigners had consequences for the health of the Japanese population. There was a dramatic increase in the incidence of cholera, dysentery, typhus, and diphtheria and it was necessary for official measures to be invoked and administrative reforms undertaken in order to deal with them. Starting with the Smallpox Prevention Regulations of 1876 the Meiji government issued a number of decrees designed to combat some of the more serious health threats (see Table 2.2).

Table 2.1 Number of hospitals by owners in the early Meiji period

Year	*Total*	*Government*			*Private*
		Sub-total	*National*	*Local*	
1874 (Meiji 7)	52	23	—	—	29
1875 (8)	63	41	—	—	22
1876 (9)	97	65	—	—	32
1877 (10)	159	124	12	112	35
1878 (11)	235	175	29	146	60
1879 (12)	309	219	42	177	90
1880 (13)	363	241	28	213	122
1881 (14)	510	335	29	306	175
1882 (15)	626	330	—	—	296
1883 (16)	—	—	—	—	—
1888*(21)	556	225	—	—	339
1889 (22)	573	222	—	—	351
1890 (23)	577	214	—	—	363
1891 (24)	579	197	—	—	382
1892 (25)	576	198	—	—	378
1893 (26)	579	198	2	106	382
1894 (27)	597	189	2	187	408
1895 (28)	589	174	2	172	415
1896 (29)	592	166	2	164	426
1897 (30)	624	159	3	156	465
1898 (31)	654	136	3	133	518

Source: Japan Ministry of Health and Welfare, *History of Medical Care for Eighty Years from the Medical Law*, 1955, p. 818
Note: *Figures from 1883 to 1887 are unavailable.

1890-1930: Industrialization, social problems, and socialization of medical care

It was only in 1889 that Japan's first modern constitution was formally promulgated by Emperor Meiji; in 1890 the first election of members to the House of Representatives took place.

As an integral part of Japan's programme of modernization government policy was to encourage and support the development of light industries such as textiles, where the start-up costs, development of facilities, acquisition of raw materials, and so on were relatively low. These industries could be quickly established moreover, thus enabling Japan to catch up with and more quickly compete with the developed countries of Europe. Government policy was manifestly successful and by the last decade of the nineteenth century Japan's first industrial revolution was nearly complete. After the Sino-Japanese War of 1894–5 and the Russo-Japanese War of 1904–5 Japan's heavy industries grew in strength and the second industrial

Table 2.2 Acute infectious disease control programmes in the early Meiji period

1871	Regulations concerning the vaccination office
1876	Smallpox Prevention Regulations
1877	Directions for Prevention of Cholera
1878	Drinking Water Warning Law
1879	Provisional Regulations for Prevention of Cholera (Establishment of Central and Local Health Councils; Health Section established in all prefectures); Seaport Cholera Infection Prevention regulations; Quarantine Regulations
1880	Epidemic Prevention Regulations
1885	Vaccination Regulations
1890	Directions for Train Quarantine
1895	Organization of Temporary Quarantine Bureau and Temporary Quarantine Department
1896	Organization of Vaccine Lymph Institute
1897	Infectious Disease Prevention Law
1899	Seaport Quarantine Law (Establishment of Seaport Quarantine Station and of Institute for Research in Infectious Diseases); Organization of Temporary Plague Prevention Office
1905	Partial Amendment to Infectious Disease Prevention Law (Liability to exterminate rats)
1909	Smallpox Vaccination Law

Source: F. Ohtani, *One Hundred Years of Health Progress in Japan*, Tokyo, International Medical Foundation of Japan, 1977, p. 36.

revolution in the country was well under way by the start of the First World War in 1914.

The economic benefits of industrialization did not immediately trickle down to the majority of the population; living conditions in the rapidly expanding urban centres were poor and the health status of the population was appalling. Japan's new cadre of western-trained physicians was growing in both size and prestige and they capitalized on their newly acquired social prominence by charging whatever fees they could for their services. The vast majority of the population could rarely afford to see one of the 'western' medical doctors. Economic and social conditions were favourable to the growth of the labour movement and socialism was winning new adherents; popular feeling against the government, a mixture of anger and fear, peaked in 1910 when a group of socialists was arrested on suspicion of regicide; after a brief and secret trial the 'conspirators' were executed.

Various significant developments were taking place in medical education which were to exert a long-lasting influence on the provision of medical care. In 1893 the departmental or 'Koza' system was implemented at Tokyo Imperial University, including the medical school. All twenty-three medical departments were to be headed by

Japanese professors who had been trained by German experts. This clearly marked the first step on the road to independence for medical education in the country. It also inaugurated a rigid vertical hierarchy, headed by an elite group of Tokyo University professors which was in many respects a re-creation of the feudal system of times gone by, compounded with German autocratic characteristics.

The second Imperial University was founded in 1897 in Kyoto where the medical school was opened two years later. Three more Imperial Universities were to be set up: the Tohoku Imperial University in 1907, the Kyushu Imperial University in 1918, and the Hokkaido Imperial University and each one eventually included a medical school.

The University Ordinance of 1918 authorized the establishment of more universities throughout the country and also approved the elevation of existing colleges and technical or vocational institutes to the status of university. The Osaka Prefectural Medical School and the Aichi Prefectural Medical School acquired university status in 1919 and 1920 respectively and were later to be merged with the Osaka and Nagoya Imperial Universities. By the end of the 1920s the majority of the former technical schools for the training of medical practitioners had been granted university status. Also in 1920 the Academic Degree Ordinance was revised to allow universities other than the Imperial Universities to award postgraduate degrees. The doctoral system together with the departmental system had the effect of strengthening the authoritarian power of the professors, because from this time onwards large numbers of medical graduates undertook postgraduate research for reasons of social prestige as much as for the purpose of obtaining further medical training.

Socialization of the medical care payment system[22-6]

Thanks to government initiatives and legislative support the medical education system developed rapidly, as did the private medical care delivery system. Payment for services was not regulated in any way and doctors could charge their patients any fees that they wished. The feudal tradition of paying for medical services in kind (e.g. rice or firewood) continued for some time after the Meiji Restoration but with the modernization of the Japanese economy, payment in cash quickly became the norm. Charges for services were raised as the growing numbers of private practitioners took advantage of increasing popular demand for their services and attempted to provide their clinics with modern equipment and to dispense the latest medication. The matter of medical fees became one of concern. In 1911 after the notorious 'High Treason' case which we referred to earlier the Emperor issued an Imperial rescript on charity medical care. He expressed his deep concern for the poor who could not afford to buy medicine or see a doctor and he donated 1.5 million yen from his private purse to the state; with a further 24 million yen collected by public subscription the government set up an Imperial charitable foundation known as the Saiseikai, which would own and operate charity clinics and welfare institutions. The Saiseikai started work in 1912 with five clinics and one visiting medical unit. By 1936 it was running fifteen hospitals, three sanatoria, one maternity hospital, sixty-one clinics and ten visiting medical units, twelve mobile nurses units, and one nursery throughout the country. Those wishing to use the facilities were given medical coupons which were issued only after some rigorous means-testing. The potential for the Saiseikai to develop into a really large-scale provider of medical care was soon limited however, first because inflation soon led to a depletion of its financial resources. Second, popular notions about 'charity' and the stigma of relying on free medical care and the humiliation of means-testing restricted the numbers of potential users.

A second development in the provision of socialized medical care also started in 1911 when a doctor called Tokijiro Kato together with an ex-businessman and a parliamentarian called Umeshiro Suzuki set up a chain of so-called thrifty medical clinics. Charges for services at these clinics were very low and the operators hoped to make them financially viable by aiming for a high turnover of patients – 'small profits and quick returns'. The clinics soon had a lot of support, especially among the working classes, and it seemed at one point that the movement would develop into quite a force in the provision of medical care in the country. However the local medical associations were opposed to the further development of such clinics and when later there was some conflict between Kato and Suzuki, the two founders, about how the network should develop, the movement eventually fell apart. The clinics had been highly successful at providing large groups of the population with medical care for moderate charges and certainly paved the way for the organization of medical co-ops and prepared the ground for the introduction of health insurance.

The first Health Insurance Law and its predecessors

Individual and small-scale efforts to provide inexpensive medical care such as we have described above could have only limited impact and government intervention was necessary for the proper organization of a social insurance scheme. In this the government had the support of the country's industrial leaders who, like the politicians, were aware of the political advantages of making some concessions to the increasingly restive socialist movement in the country in the first two decades of the twentieth century. Japan's first health insurance law was therefore passed by the Diet in 1922, its enactment was delayed until 1926, and the payment of benefits actually got under way in 1927. The 1922 Act was preceded by several proposals and individual initiatives to develop insurance-based schemes of medical care financing for the population. One of the most enlightened and eager proponents of social health insurance was Shinpei Goto (1857–1929) who started as an office boy at a prefectural government office as a 13-year-old, later studied at medical school, and eventually became a hospital administrator; he was later appointed to a series of increasingly important government posts including Director of the Bureau of Health at the Home Ministry, a senior position in the Government-General of Taiwan, President of the Manchurian Railways, Minister of Posts and Telecommunications, Minister of Foreign Affairs, Mayor of Tokyo and the Minister of Home Affairs. He had been sent to Germany from 1889 to 1892 and took the opportunity to observe the organization and operation of German social insurance schemes which had been introduced in the 1880s. On his return to Japan he assiduously promoted the concept of social insurance, particularly health insurance, during the 1890s, as he was convinced of its importance in the protection and maintenance of a sound labour force as well as its role in keeping industrial peace. His ideas were perhaps too advanced to receive much hearing among his government colleagues and the industrial leaders of the day.

But some action was being taken; mutual aid associations were organized at Ani Mine in Akita in 1888, at a cement company in Yamaguchi in 1889, and at the Kanebo Textile Company in 1905, all of which can be considered as pioneers in the private sector. In the government sector, mutual aid associations were set up at Yawata Iron Work Corporation in 1905 and at the Imperial Railways Agency in 1907. From then until the early 1920s other mutual aid associations were organized at the Government Monopoly Agency, the Government Printing Office, the Postal and Telecommunications Corporation, the Navy Ministry, the Army Ministry, the Forestry Agency, the Police Agency and the Government Mint. It is sometimes said that the Health Insurance Bill sneaked through the Diet in the shadows of, and overshadowed by, the contentious debates which attended the passing of the Peace Regulation Bill in 1925 which took the nation into the 'dark valley' of the 1930s.

The main features of Japan's Health Insurance Law were the provision of medical treatment for disease, injuries, and death (including those related to work or childbirth) and some cash allowances. Provision of benefits was limited to a maximum 180-day period and only the insured individual was covered. Employees whose annual wage was less than 1,200 yen and who worked more than 120 successive days at factories and mines covered by the Factory Act or the Mining Act were compulsorily insured. Employees at any work-place with fewer than five employees were to be voluntarily insured. In principle the government was to manage health insurance; however, private firms with 300 or more employees were allowed to set up individual health insurance societies. Thus were the beginnings of the separation and segmentation of Japan's health insurance system which still applies today. Individual employees were required to make a contribution proportional to their wage or salary and some of the contribution was picked up by their employers. Although the Health Insurance Law was a definite advance it was a limited piece of legislation and was not without its problems. Because of the in-built restriction on income and size of work-place fewer than 2 million out of an estimated 4.7 million workers in the country were eligible for compulsory insurance. The largest numbers excluded were to be found among the employees of small workshops and family enterprises where conditions were particularly poor. Industrial accidents and injuries and work-related diseases once compensated by employers were now covered by the new insurance benefits but many workers fell outside the health insurance scheme. Such workers now had to meet medical costs themselves; consequently and perhaps not surprisingly they bitterly attacked the legislation. Total income, including different allowances, was the basis of calculation of each employee's contribution which became relatively high and represented a new and unavoidable financial burden for many families. Exclusion of dependants was clearly also a disadvantage.

Reaction to the health insurance system varied. Industrialists were uneasy about the availability of free medical care and cash allowances and were concerned that the system would be abused and productivity would decline. Employers in the small and medium-sized companies complained about the burden of their contributions to employee health insurance. The physicians were unhappy about the low rate of fees paid under health insurance; the workers themselves were not happy with a system which seemed to be distinguished by so many gaps and limitations. Under the leadership of an extremely radical Marxist Labour Union Council, organized in 1925, an anti-health insurance strike was organized and affected the majority of the country's mines and factories. This strike marked something of a turning-point in the history of Japanese unionism and labour relations; none the less the provisions of the Health Insurance Law went through and payment of benefits started in 1927.

Official measures for the prevention of specific diseases[27,28]

By the end of the nineteenth century the government had in place various measures designed to control the spread of a number of acute infectious diseases which had been growing in incidence and prevalence since the opening up of the country some forty years earlier. In the first two decades of the twentieth century official attention focused on several chronic diseases which had long been found in the country but which had become more prominent as she modernized and industrialized. The government was often slow to tackle problems as it was mindful of the needs of the country's industrialists and tended to implement much-needed reforms and legislation only when the health status of the military was seriously threatened or affected. Specific diseases which attracted public concern were venereal diseases, leprosy, mental disorders, tuberculosis, silicosis, beriberi, trachoma, and some particularly dreadful parasitic diseases endemic to the country.

Venereal diseases Cases of VD were first recorded in Japan in 1515 and the disease spread quickly across the country. After the Meiji Restoration VD spread particularly quickly and just as the phrase 'Civilization is syphilization' might have been an appropriate catchphrase for the Renaissance in Europe so too might it have described the Meiji era in Japan. In the early 1880s it was reported that at the health inspection for conscripts about two-thirds of examinees suffered from VD. Table 2.3 illustrates the high number of VD hospitals in the Meiji era.

Officially permitted red-light districts were common in most Japanese cities during the Edo era and the prostitutes were usually girls from poor families who had been sold off to brothels as a

Table 2.3 Numbers of hospitals in the early Meiji period

Year	*Total number*	*Hospitals*	*Branch hospitals*	*Insane asylums*	*VD hospitals*	*Beriberi hospitals*	*Leper houses*	*Others*
1875	63	59	—	—	3	—	—	1
1876	97	89	—	—	7	—	—	1
1877	159	146	—	—	12	—	—	1
1878	235	124	63	1	40	—	4	3
1879	309	165	71	3	61	—	6	3
1880	363	234	55	3	57	3	6	5
1881	510	281	73	5	135	4	5	7
1882	626	402	64	6	130	5	5	14

Source: Japan Ministry of Health and Welfare, *Eighty Years of Medical Care in Japan*, (Isei 80 Nenshi), Government Printing Office, Tokyo, 1955, p. 82.

means of raising money for the family. The system continued under the Meiji government and was not in fact repealed until 1956, when the Anti-Prostitution Law came into force. A system of inspection of prostitutes was originated after a request from a Russian Admiral in Nagasaki in 1860, whose crew members were allowed ashore while their damaged vessel was undergoing repairs. The inspections were organized by Pompe van Meerdervoort, whose students carried them out. Similar checks were organized in Yokohama in 1867 for British soldiers after a request by the British Minister Parks. In 1867 the system was expanded to cover the whole country. Records of the day showed the following statistics: in 1878 65.1 per cent of employed prostitutes were infected with VD. By 1883 75.8 per cent were infected and by 1888 92 per cent of those checked were found to have the disease. Under the Prostitutes Control Law of 1900 the inspection of prostitutes became compulsory and this law undoubtedly contributed to the continuation of an officially sanctioned system. Many physicians also favoured the system, as they considered that it helped to limit the spread of venereal disease. Equally, other community groups argued against the system on the grounds that the officially permitted brothels simply became the seed beds for further infection. The system was also opposed on the grounds that it was an official violation of women's rights. However as the opposition was led by minority Christian missionary groups the government was able to ignore it for some time. One prefecture, Gunma, was rather more radical and had abolished officially sanctioned prostitution as early as 1894; the ratio of VD patients fell below the national average and results of health examinations for conscripts improved significantly, as we can see in Tables 2.4 and 2.5. Further legislation was in the Venereal Disease Prevention Law of 1927.

Leprosy Lepers traditionally suffered vicious discrimination in Japan; rejected by their families and community they were condemned to a life as wandering beggars or vagabond pilgrims. Temples and shrines were well-known gathering places for lepers: some organized loosely knit communities well away from the villages and communities. In the early days of the Meiji Restoration foreigners were particularly appalled by the conditions of the lepers; their official complaints to the authorities caused the Japanese government some considerable shame and embarrassment. Several private 'leprosaria' had been set up in the middle of the nineteenth century and in the last decade of the century foreign Christian missionary groups established and ran another group of facilities. Knowledge about the disease was limited and the treatment at the

Table 2.4 Ratio of VD patients at the age of conscription exams in Gunma Prefecture and Japan (per 1,000)

Year	*Gunma Prefecture*	*All Japan*
1921	11.13	18.71
1922	10.67	17.46
1923	18.06	15.23
1924	15.27	15.23
1925	11.73	13.78
1926	11.46	13.28
1927	7.63	11.85
Average	12.27	14.93

Source: K. Maruyama, *Medical History in Gunma Prefecture* (Gunma no Ishi), Gunma Prefectural Medical Association, 1958, p. 337.

Table 2.5 Ratio of VD patients at the age of conscription exams in Gunma Prefecture by residents and non-residents (per 1,000)

Year	*Resident in Gunma*	*Non-resident*
1923	10.01	174.32
1924	9.67	123.82
1925	8.21	90.32
1926	7.72	90.71
1927	4.21	73.50
Average	7.89	112.08

Source: K. Maruyama, *Medical History in Gunma Prefecture* (Gunma no Ishi), Gunma Prefectural Medical Association, 1958, p. 337.

leprosaria or at the dermatology departments of university and other hospitals was not of the best. The use of quack drugs which came and went at the whim of fashion did nothing to help the sufferers and their numbers within the community did not decline, much to the annoyance and anger of officialdom. The government took radical action finally in 1907 with the Lepers Control Regulation. This law established five public regional leprosaria and empowered local authorities to detain homeless lepers compulsorily. Administration of the leprosy control act rested with the police who had similar powers for the control of acute infectious diseases. Because leprosy was not curable and treatment ineffective those sufferers who were detained were essentially condemned to a life-long jail sentence in the leprosaria which were strictly run and offered little therapy for the residents. Many became mentally ill and attempts at escape were frequent. In 1931 the 1907 Regulation was revised and the Leprosy

Prevention Law provided for free in-patient care for all leprosy patients at national government-run facilities.

Mentally ill people[27,29] In a society which emphasizes and promotes conformity to the norm mentally ill people are doubly disadvantaged. Japan has historically paid scant regard to the welfare and rights of mentally ill or handicapped people. In feudal times mentally ill people were sent to prison or banished to prison islands. Up until the early years of the Meiji era mentally ill people could be arrested and tried for any crime. The Criminal Law of 1880 provided for the first time that crimes arising from mental disturbance could not be punished. This was a remarkable step forward in Japanese legal and medical history but real implementation of the law was sporadic and unreliable partly because expert doctors were not always available for judgement or diagnosis. Most mentally ill patients were condemned to a miserable existence either at asylums or in their own homes and they were often handcuffed, fettered, locked away, and neglected. From the early years of the Meiji Restoration the supervision of mental patients was under the control of the police authorities, who could authorize their detention at home if relatives notified them that a family member was showing 'abnormal' behaviour. This provision was designed to ensure public order and security and did not have in mind the welfare and rights of mentally ill or handicapped people. In 1901, when Dr Shuzo Kure came back from Germany and was appointed Professor of Psychiatry at the Tokyo Imperial University Medical School as well as director of a Tokyo mental hospital, there came the beginning of some moderate improvements in the lot of mental patients in Japan. Dr Kure prohibited the use of fetters and other restraints on mental patients and finally ordered the destruction of such equipment. This was more than one hundred years after Phillipe Pinel (1745–1826) had unchained mental patients in Paris at the time of the French Revolution.

Dr Kure also carried out a comprehensive survey, 'The Situation of Mental Patients Confined at their Homes', from 1910 to 1916 in Tokyo and fourteen other prefectures. In his findings (published in 1918) Dr Kure noted that the total number of beds at mental hospitals was 5,000 for the whole of the country and he estimated the total number of patients at between 140,000 and 150,000, so approximately 3.5 per cent of mental patients could be accommodated at purpose-built hospitals. The remaining number of mentally ill patients could be divided into three groups according to the type of accommodation. The first group comprised members of wealthy families or the less seriously ill who were treated in general

Figure 2.1 Tuberculosis death-rates in selected countries, 1900–73

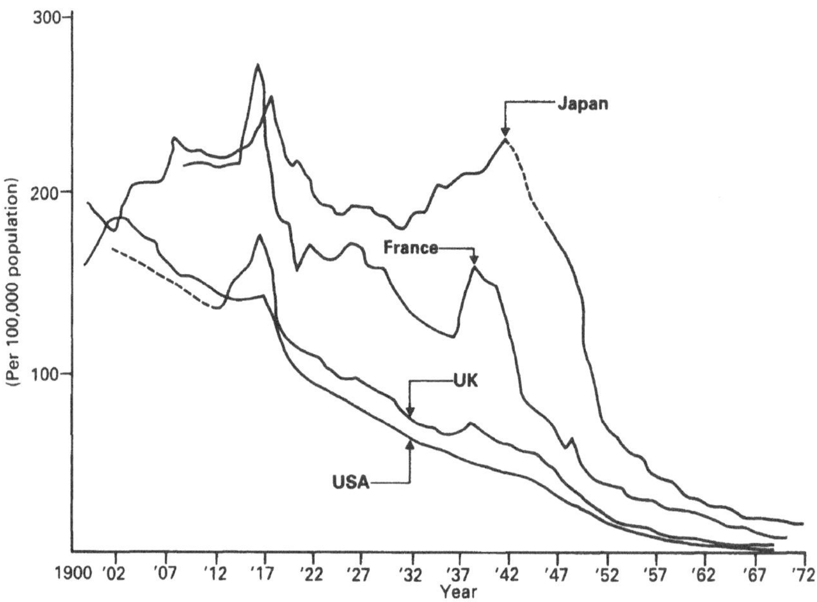

Source: Statistics of Information Department, Ministry of Health and Welfare, Tokyo, 1987

medical facilities or cared for at home. The second group were usually chained for confinement at home. The third group were treated at shrines and temples for faith-healing. The second and third groups constituted the majority and were the prime focus of Dr Kure's research; he was concerned particularly to improve the lot of those people who were confined within their own homes. Dr Kure had to conclude at the end of all his work that the treatment of mentally ill people in Japan was appalling and far behind that of western countries; it led him to consider too that mentally ill people in Japan were unhappy not only because of their illness but also because they were Japanese.

Tuberculosis[27] Tuberculosis had been common in Japan for many years before the modern period but its incidence increased dramatically at the beginning of the twentieth century and its growth was associated with poor living and working conditions as the country underwent rapid urbanization and industrialization. Figure 2.1 illustrates the trend in mortality rates for tuberculosis in Japan compared to rates in the UK, the USA, and France. The surge in

Table 2.6 Numbers and ratios of workers by sex, 1894–1918 (1,000s)

Year	*Male workers*	*Female workers*	*Proportion female workers*
1894	141.9	239.4	62.7
1896	173.6	261.2	60.0
1899	158.8	264.4	64.8
1902	185.6	313.3	62.8
1905	240.3	347.6	59.1
1908	248.8	400.9	61.7
1913	375.5	540.6	59.0
1918	646.1	763.0	54.2

Source: M. Kiichi, *Nihon Rodosha Kaikyu Jotaishi*, Tokyo: Sonichi Shobo, 1961, p. 44.

the spread of tuberculosis in Japan was aided by a chain that went from factory girls to farming communities and then on to soldiers. As already mentioned, Japan's initial industrialization was in the light industries such as textiles which depended heavily on cheap labour. At the same time heavy land taxes were impoverishing many rural families and communities who survived only by sending their daughters to the cities to work in the textile mills. Conditions were very harsh, the working day long, and even in their free time the girls were strictly supervised and made to live in dormitories. Their pathetic existence became a matter of public scandal after the publication of various personal stories in the press and reports by government inspectors highlighted the grimness of their lives. Table 2.6 shows that female factory workers constituted more than half of the labour force in the first two decades of the twentieth century.

The tuberculosis 'chain' went into operation when female factory workers, worn-out and ill, returned to their native villages where the population was not immunized and therefore susceptible to catching the disease. Immediate family members were the first to catch the disease and it would soon spread around the rest of the community. As the rural communities were a major source of supply of soldiers, tuberculosis thus became a serious problem for the army authorities. Table 2.7 illustrates trends in the numbers of tuberculosis sufferers among discharged soldiers.

The government was forced eventually to take some action about this very real health problem and the Factory Bill of 1900 was designed to enforce some improvements in working conditions; however massive opposition from powerful industrialists meant that the Bill did not actually get through the Diet until 1911. A hygienist, Dr Osamu Ishihara, did an excellent survey on 'Female factory workers and tuberculosis', the results of which shocked the public

Table 2.7 Ratio of discharged soldiers with TB (per 10,000)

Year	%
1887	7.7
1888	8.6
1889	9.8
1890	13.9
1891	17.0
1892	20.6
1893	20.6
1894	—
1895	—
1896	22.2
1897	23.5
1898	33.6
1899	38.0
1900	41.4

Source: Japan Institute of Public Health, *Koshueisei no Hattatsu*, 1967, p. 487

when they were published in 1913. He described in detail the horrendous living and working conditions of female factory workers and presented his theory on the spread of tuberculosis from the girls to the rest of the community. He analysed mortality rates for females in the same age groups among the community at large and among factory workers and concluded that the deaths of 5,000 female workers annually could be directly attributed to their occupation. He suggested that the responsible industrialists were guilty *de facto* of murder and yet they had managed to avoid any punishment. His work and findings eventually secured political support; the Factory Act finally came into force in 1916. It prescribed an eleven-hour working day for women and children, and a minimum age of 12 years.

During this period there were other pieces of legislation aimed at controlling the spread of tuberculosis, for example the Cattle Tuberculosis Prevention Law of 1901. In 1904 the Ordinance on Tuberculosis Prevention called for the provision of spittoons, disinfection of sputa in public places, and the disinfection of tuberculosis patients' homes and property. The Tuberculosis Law of 1919 amalgamated earlier legislation and provided for disinfection, government subsidies to local governments, and semi-public organizations running sanatoria. The only treatment available at the time was fresh air, rest, and improved nutrition; different medication, some useful, some not, was also tried with varying results. It was only after the Second World War that the disease was finally completely controlled.

Silicosis, endemic parastic diseases, beriberi, and trachoma[27,30] These illustrate a range of occupational, locality-determined, and nation-wide diseases which had long afflicted the people of Japan. Silicosis was an 'old' occupational disease among the country's mineworkers and they had organized local mutual aid associations throughout the country. Before the real cause of schistosoma japonicum and other parasitic diseases was discovered, many believed that they were genetic and patients and their families consequently suffered considerable discrimination in their communities.

Beriberi and trachoma were widely prevalent and because large numbers of soldiers were affected the government and military authorities were eventually forced to do something. Beriberi was initially thought to be an acute infectious disease because it seemed to affect large numbers of people who showed acute symptoms. It caused the same level of fear among the Japanese as did cholera in Europe. The incidence of the disease did take on epidemic proportions in the Edo era as the Japanese started to eat more highly polished rice and the urban areas of Edo (Tokyo), Osaka, and Kyoto were particularly affected. After the Meiji Restoration the incidence of beriberi increased dramatically and in 1877 the government ordered public hospitals to report on the number of cases encountered, on symptoms, therapies and the findings of autopsies. According to an annual report of the Health Bureau of the Home Ministry, from January to June 1879 in Tokyo and twenty-four prefectures (a total population of 22,033,577) there were 3,170 beriberi patients of whom 391 died, a mortality rate of 12.3 per cent. In 1878 a government-sponsored specialist beriberi hospital was built and practitioners of western medicine and traditional Chinese medicine vied with each other to see which system of treatment was the most effective. As neither approach dealt with the underlying cause of the disease the competition naturally ended in a stalemate. With the expansion of the military forces, the incidence of beriberi in the armed forces became serious. In 1878 approximately one-third of all soldiers were found to be suffering from a form of the disease and the mortality rate was approximately 30 per cent. In the navy Dr Kanehiro Takagi, director of the Navy Hospital in Tokyo, who had come back from Britain in 1880, insisted that the staple food be changed from polished rice to a mixture of rice and barley. His recommendations were vindicated when incidence of the disease fell rapidly in the navy. In the army, however, high-ranking surgeons stuck to the theories emanating from Germany that beriberi was an infectious disease and thus would not concede the obviously beneficial affects of the mixed rice and barley-meal diet in the prevention of the disease. (Writing in 1881 Mary Crawford Fraser, wife of the British Minister (Ambassador), noted that 'kakke' or beriberi was unknown in her amah's province because a kind of oatmeal was mixed with the rice. And further, 'The soldiers suffer from it a good deal; but it is hoped that the meat diet lately introduced in alternation with the native rice and fish food will do much to overcome the weakness. In the navy the men are generously fed on meat, rather to their distaste, but very much to their physical well-being'.) In 1911 Dr Umetaro Suzuki reported on his discovery of a previously unknown nutritive element in the rice bran and named it 'Oryzanin' and concluded that its absence in the diet was possibly related to the incidence of beriberi. His discovery was more or less ignored by Japanese medical circles. In the following year Casimir Funk (1884–1967) working independently extracted the same substance and named it vitamin (thiamine). His findings were accepted in the west and it was eventually recognized in Japan that Oryzanin and thiamine were the same substance. Once the cause of beriberi was clearly established official preventive measures were implemented and the disease has been virtually unknown in Japan since the 1920s.

1930–45 The road to war and its impact on developments in medical care[7,31-3]

By the end of the First World War Japan had achieved many of the social, political, and economic goals which the leaders of the Meiji Restoration had set for her. The war itself had contributed significantly to the growth in the country's economy, which was now highly developed, more than matched her military might, and certainly enhanced her growing stature as a world power. Textiles and light industry continued to account for a large proportion of her export trade but heavy industry had also matured and Japan was now producing much of her own industrial machinery and equipment and was rapidly expanding her shipbuilding capacity. Japan's industrial development was notable for the parallel growth of two distinct kinds of industrial organization – which still exist today. On the one hand were the massive, multi-sectoral conglomerates: the 'zaibatsu', which were involved in everything from heavy industry, iron and steel, shipbuilding, to banking, trading, and commerce, which could because of their very nature protect themselves in times of economic recession. On the other hand there were the small, usually family-owned and operated enterprises which concentrated on the manufacture of necessary components and parts. But Japan soon felt the effects of the post-war trade depression; the 1923 earthquake which devastated Tokyo drained resources and slowed down growth. A banking crisis in 1927 bankrupted many small firms but contributed to a strengthening of the economic might and enhanced the political sway of the 'zaibatsu'. Inflation affected all sectors of society and unrest in the cities eventually spread to the countryside which for some time had been relatively protected. The Japanese people after the First World War were undoubtedly better fed, housed, and clothed than before it, and in the cities many could enjoy the new amenities such as electricity, radio, and access to books and newspapers. But not everyone benefited from the country's overall prosperity and for many cogs in the industrial machine life was unmitigated misery and hardship. In the countryside too the poorer farmers and tenant farmers eventually had to absorb the impact of industrial recession as people who had migrated to the cities to work in the new factories were forced to return to their villages when they were unemployed. It is noteworthy that the core of the Japanese army came from the peasantry and many of the officers came from the small and medium landowning families who were particularly conservative. Officers of this type were shocked by the amount and depth of corruption among politicians and despised their collusion with the 'zaibatsu' for their own political and financial gain. Fanatic ultra-nationalistic ideas on how to rebuild Japan prevailed in the 1930s and inspired the younger army officers especially. By a combination of unchecked aggression abroad and murderous conspiracy at home extremists in the military gradually started to exert control over a weak and leaderless government.

In 1928 officers of the Kwantung Army – the Japanese garrison in southern Manchuria – assassinated the Chinese warlord of Manchuria, Chang Tsao-Lin; in 1931 it made attacks on the railways in Manchuria and claimed that these were guerrilla attacks by the Chinese and thus provoked the Japanese into seizing control of the Province. The 'Manchuria Incident' marked the beginning of the fifteen years' war between Japan and China and set Japan on the road to her involvement in the Second World War.

The 1930s were a time of political tension and upheaval in the country. Growing militarism gave a new significance to the need for a strong and healthy military. The health status of the Japanese people was, however, deteriorating as shown by the deplorable records of health examinations for conscription, the high and growing incidence of tuberculosis, and the abysmal infant mortality-rate statistics. For those without insurance – the majority – medical care was expensive, if indeed a doctor was available. Many areas were without adequate doctors, clinics, or hospitals. The market principle of medical care was encouraged by the government and did not foster equitable distribution of services or facilities.

The early 1930s saw two notable attempts to change the existing provisions and to develop socialized medical care. One was the movement for the development of co-operative medical care facilities, led by famous Christian intellectuals such as Toyohiko Kagawa and Inazo Nitobe. Then there was the socialist or communist movement for medical care facilities for workers and farmers, initiated in memory of Senji Yamamoto, a Communist member of the Diet who had been opposed to the Maintenance of Public Order Bill, had been an early supporter of birth control, and had been assassinated by a fanatic nationalist youth in 1929. A chain of hospitals and clinics was developed throughout the country; at one time there were some twenty such facilities for farmers and workers, but their sponsorship by the Communists was unacceptable to the authorities and the facilities were eventually closed down by the police. The last such clinic, in Niigata, was closed down in 1941. The movement was revived after the Second World War as the 'Democratic Medical Facility Movement' and in 1953 the Federation of Democratic Medical Facilities was organized. The first group we mentioned, the co-operative movement, merged with other groups such as the agricultural co-operative association and expanded. Some of the movement's associated facilities were taken over during the war by the Japan Medical Corporation, the official body in charge of wartime medical care services. The Japan Medical Corporation was dissolved at the end of the war and the co-operative medical care facilities were absorbed into the mainstream medical care delivery system.

More direct government intervention to improve the medical care delivery system resulted from strong pressure from the military authorities during the mid-1930s. Under the National Health Insurance Act of 1938 a national health insurance society was to be organized in each municipality to cover self-employed people such as farmers and fishermen and their families and thus to make medical care more accessible to them. In the same year the Ministry of Health and Welfare was established as an independent health and social welfare authority from the Home Ministry.

The Health Centre Act of 1937 called for the opening of public health centres, part of the government's policy of having 'Healthy People, Healthy Soldiers', and by 1938 the centres were starting to operate and offered preventive health services, health education, and guidance. The National Institute of Public Health was opened in 1938 to train public health personnel. The building of the Institute was financed by donations from the Rockefeller Foundation.

With the beginning of the Pacific War on 8 December 1941 (Japan time: 7 December in the USA and Europe) the country came under total wartime conditions. In 1942 the National Medical Service Act regulated on all matters relating to the medical and health professions and set up the Japan Medical Corporation, which was charged with the development and organization of a nation-wide network of medical facilities. The Japan Medical Corporation Plan called for two central hospitals with 500 beds each: one in Tokyo to serve the north-eastern half of the country and one in Osaka for the south-western half. There were to be 47 prefectural hospitals with 250 beds each and 588 district hospitals with 50 beds each; clinics or surgeries were to be established in communities without doctors by building new facilities or commandeering other available public facilities and converting them. In addition to this public network for general medical care services, 100,000 new beds in tuberculosis sanatoria were to be developed. The underlying concepts of the systematic planning, organization, and administration of health care provisions inaugurated by the Japan Medical Corporation were similar to the proposals of the Dawson Report of 1920 in Britain which was to provide the foundation for the National Health Service established in 1948.

The Japan Medical Corporation was dissolved by the Occupying Forces in 1947; at that time it had 20 prefectural hospitals, 198 district hospitals, 282 clinics, 5 maternity hospitals, 87 tuberculosis sanatoria, and 96 convalescent homes, a total of 688 facilities, under its authority. All these facilities were returned to their previous owners or transferred to different organizations. The wartime effort of the Japan Medical Corporation to establish a unified and public health care delivery system ended half-way. It is supposed however that even after the country's defeat officials of the Ministry of Health and Welfare were nostalgic for the rational planning of the country's health care delivery system which had prevailed during wartime; several recommendations issued in the immediate post-war years proposed that the rehabilitation of Japan's medical facilities should be based on a public sector oriented model. Then in 1959 a blueprint for a nation-wide pyramidal medical care delivery network was drawn up by the Ministry of Health and Welfare, but had to be shelved in the face of massive opposition from the free-market oriented Japan Medical Association, which was growing more powerful and condemned the proposals as militaristic nostalgia on the part of ministry officials. The preparation and submission of a regional medical plan for each prefecture required under the 1985 amendments to the Medical Service Law may mark at last the realization of a long-cherished dream of officials of the Ministry of Health and Welfare.

The war years saw some expansion of the health insurance systems. In 1939 dependants of the insured could take out voluntary insurance and this became compulsory in 1943. Office employees and seamen also became eligible for insurance and in 1944 the term of benefit was extended to two years from the previous 180 days. By the end of the war in 1945 approximately one-third of the population was covered by some insurance; ironically the availability of medical care was severely limited as many facilities had been destroyed by bombing, the production of drugs and other medical supplies was severely disrupted, and most male physicians had been drafted by the military. More than half of all the insurance societies were either defunct or functioning only with limited capacity.

In order to meet wartime needs for medical personnel the government had approved the three-year medical course in thirteen national medical schools in 1939. Between 1943 and 1944 thirty-one new medical schools were opened which likewise provided the short-term course of medical education. With the graduation of these physicians and the return of doctors from military service at the end of the war there were problems of over-supply and some difficulties because of differences in education and training. Those doctors who had received the short training course often experienced discrimination when it came to obtaining employment for example. As part of postwar education reforms during 1948–52 the number of medical schools was reduced from seventy-four to forty-six and all were designated as providing university-level education and training.

We have described in broad terms the major developments in the history of health and medical care in Japan and the social and political and cultural influences which have shaped its progress up until 1945.

For more than a thousand years the country relied on a system of medical care imported from her cultural mentor, China. She adapted and added to this body of knowledge, then slowly and cautiously acquired and assimilated new ideas and knowledge from the west. The vast majority of the population was unable to reap even the limited benefits of 'kampo' as its practitioners were few and they tended to restrict their practice to members of the aristocracy or the growing merchant class. With what must be considered truly incredible speed and remarkable ease Japan then replaced her traditional system of medical care and opted for western medical science. She retained some of the characteristics of what had gone before and traditional popular attitudes about the elevated status and superior knowledge of the medical practitioner were, and perhaps remain, slow to change.

In a country which seems to be permanently and voraciously bent on change, on replacing the 'old' with the newest, the present system of health and medical care is now considered, after one hundred years, to be long established, indeed 'traditional'. The western, scientific approach to medical and health care reigns supreme although there are some who are beginning to question the limitations of this approach and appreciate their fortune in having the underlying philosophy and values of the system that went before to refer to.

As for the organization of health and medical care services, we have seen how concrete political realities and goals have shaped the nature of the Japanese system to date. Government interest in the organization of health services has been rooted not only in a desire to emulate and catch up with the west (the Meiji Restoration), but also in a concern to ensure a healthy work-force to aid Japan's industrial development and to maintain her military might. By and large individuals have carried the responsibility for their health care and market forces have shaped the nature and availability of services. Attempts to develop socialized health care delivery systems have come and for the most part gone quickly! The developments which have occurred in specific areas since 1945 will form the subject-matter for the following chapters.

References

1 En-Sheng Li, personal letter, Beijing, 1985.
2 J. Cai, 'Traditional Chinese medicine and some of its social aspects', D. Wu and K. Sonodo (eds) *Proceedings for the Workshop on Modernisation of East Asian Medicine*, Honolulu, 7–19 January, 1986.
3 Y. Otsuka, 'History of Medicine', *Kodansha Encyclopedia of Japan*, Tokyo, Kodanasha, 1986, pp. 145–7.
4 A. Ishihara, *Nihon No Igaku* (Medicine in Japan), Tokyo, Shibundo, 1959.
5 R. Storry, *A History of Modern Japan*, Harmondsworth, Penguin, 1960.
6 S. Fuse, *Ishi No Rekishi* (History of Physicians), Tokyo, Chuokoronsha, 1979.
7 T. Kawakami, *Gendai Nihon Iryoshi* (History of Medicine in Modern Japan), Tokyo, Keiso Shobo, 1965.
8 T. Kawakami, 'Medical care in the capitalist society', in *Medical Care and Social Welfare*, Tokyo, Keisoshobo, 1973, pp. 181–217.
9 F. Ohtani, *On Hundred Years of Health Progress in Japan*, Tokyo, International Medical Foundation of Japan, 1971.
10 A. Sugaya, *Nihon Iryoseidoshi* (History of medical care system in Japan), Tokyo, Hara Shobo, 1976.
11 Japan Ministry of Health and Welfare, *Isei 50 Nenshi* (Fifty Years of Medical Care System in Japan), Tokyo, 1925.
12 Japan Ministry of Health and Welfare, *Isei 80 Nenshi* (Eighty Years of

Medical Care System in Japan), Tokyo, 1955.
13 Japan Ministry of Health and Welfare, *Isei 100 Nenshi* (One Hundred Years of Medical Care System in Japan), Tokyo, 1976.
14 P. Akamatsu, *Meiji 1868: Revolution and Counter Revolution in Japan*, trans. M. Kochan, London, Allen & Unwin, 1972.
15 W.G. Beasley, *The Modern History of Japan*, 3rd revised edn, Tokyo, C.E. Tuttle, 1973, p. 216.
16 H. Cortazzi, *Dr. Willis in Japan, 1862–1877. A British Medical Pioneer*, London, Athlone Press, 1985.
17 E. Baelz, *Awakening Japan: The Diary of a German Doctor*, Bloomington, Indiana, Indiana University Press, 1974.
18 A. Kamiya, *Nihon Kindai Igaku No Akebono* (The Dawn of Modern Medicine in Japan), Tokyo, Iryotoshoshuppansha, 1979.
19 M. Anesaki, 'Iikuseido wo Tooshitemita Ishi no Career Pattern to Byoin ono Kizokuishiki Keisei no Rekishiteki Gaikan' (The career pattern of Japanese physicians in relation to the medical education system), *Byoin Kanri*, 10, vol. 1, January 1972, pp. 31–8.
20 A. Sugaya, *Nihon no Byoin* (Hospitals in Japan), Tokyo, Chuokoronsha, 1981.
21 M. Anesaki, 'Byoin no Kinobunka' (Differentiation of hospital functions), *Jurist*, Special issue: Medical Care and Human Rights, November 1973, Tokyo, Yuhikaku, pp. 167–72.
22 T. Saguchi, *Nihon Shakaihokenshi* (History of Social Insurance in Japan), Tokyo, Nihonhyoronshinsha, 1957.
23 B. Kondo, *Shakaihoken* (Social Insurance), Tokyo, Iwanamishoten, 1963.
24 T. Saguchi, *Nihon no Iryohosho* (Social Security in Medical Care in Japan), Tokyo, Toyokeizaishinposha, 1966.
25 K. Ogawa (ed.), *Kenkohokenho Seiritsushi* (History of Enactment of Health Insurance Bill), Osaka Municipal University Economic society, 1974.
26 B. Kondo, *Nihon no Shakaihosho no Rekishi* (History of Social Security in Japan), Tokyo, Koseishuppansha, 1974.
27 T. Kawakami, *Gendai Nihon Byoninshi* (History of Sick People in Modern Japan), Tokyo, Keisoshobo, 1982.
28 S. Tatsukawa, *Byoki no Shakaishi* (Society History of Diseases), Tokyo, Nihon Hoso Shuppan Kyokai, 1971.
29 S. Kure *et al.* 'Seishin Byosha Shitak Kanchi no Jikkyo' (Report on detained medical patients in their houses), 'Tokyo Igakki Zasshi 32, nos 10–13, 1918.
30 M.C. Fraser, *A Diplomat's Wife in Japan*, ed. H. Cortazzi, Tokyo, Weatherhill, 1982, p. 317.
31 T. Nomura, *Kokumin no Iryoshi* (People's History of Medical Care), Tokyo, Sanseido, 1977.
32 T. Nomura, *Senjika Iryoseisaku Shusei* (Collection of Medical Care Policy Documents in Wartime), Tokyo, Iryotosho Shuppansha, 1978.
33 T. Nomura, *Iryo to Kokuminseikatsu* (Medical Care and People's Lives), Tokyo, Aokishoten, 1981.

Chapter three

Patterns and trends in mortality and morbidity

We noted briefly in the previous chapter some of the important epidemiological trends in Japan from earliest times through to the period of modernization in the nineteenth century and then on to her defeat in the Second World War. In this chapter we look at the principal patterns of disease and causes of death in the 1980s and we highlight some of the changes that have taken place in the past forty years, changes which have had influence on, and will continue to influence the country's health services into the next century.

Demographic changes

Ironically Christianity was one of the reasons why the Japanese first made a serious attempt at counting themselves. The country's first reliable attempt at a census took place in 1721 and was aimed partly at rooting out any left-over Christians in the population at large, Christianity having been officially banned some 130 years earlier. The system of family registers was gradually developed by the Tokugawa authorities and they conducted a count of the population every six years until 1852.[1] After four years in office the Meiji government held its first, and only, census (in 1872) in order to set up a complete family registration system; in fact these family registers provided a reasonably accurate reckoning of births, deaths, and marriages at community level throughout the country until the first full-scale modern census of the population was carried out in 1920. Censuses now take place every ten years.

According to estimates from the Edo period Japan's population stayed at a fairly constant 30–32 million people from 1721 to the late nineteenth century. The country had a high birth-rate but population growth was kept down, thanks to late marriage and a high death-rate, the latter caused by frequent famines, natural disasters, and recurrent epidemics of infectious diseases. It is thought too that induced abortion and the practice of infanticide were fairly widespread throughout the society.

The census of 1872 estimated the country's population at 34.8 million. It grew to 42 million by 1896, 47 million by 1906, and 50 million by 1912. With a total of 70 million people in 1940 we can see that the Japanese population had doubled in just over seventy years. Throughout the 1930s the country had experienced high birth-rates but death-rates were beginning to decline slowly, thanks to economic growth and the associated improvements in living conditions and health care. The population therefore grew at a steady rate during the 1920s and 1930s; the 1940s saw much greater fluctuations – the population decreased in the first half of the decade, because of the war, and shot up in the second half of the decade. Both the birth-rate and death-rate dropped considerably in the 1950s and total population growth fell to rates comparable to those in the western industrial countries. The country had 104.7 million people in 1970 and in 1986, with a population of 122 million, Japan was the seventh-largest nation in the world, and exhibited the low birth- and death-rates characteristic of a country which had completed the demographic transition (see Table 3.1). Indeed Japan is the only non-European country to have done so since the Second World War.

Table 3.1 World population ranking (estimates of mid-year population, 1984)

Country	*Ranking*	*Estimated population* (10,000s)
China	1	105,155
India	2	74,674
USSR	3	27,500
USA	4	23,668
Indonesia	5	15,989
Brazil	6	13,258
Japan	7	12,002
Bangladesh	8	9,673
Pakistan	9	9,329
Nigeria	10	9,204

Source: UN Demographic Yearbook, 1984

We can see more details of Japan's population growth from 1872 as well as projections of her population growth until 2080 in Figure 3.1 and Table 3.2.

Birth-rates and fertility decline

Birth-rates in the early years of Meiji were very high and a figure of 32 births per 1,000 population was recorded for 1900; in the first

Figure 3.1 Population growth and population projections, 1872–2080

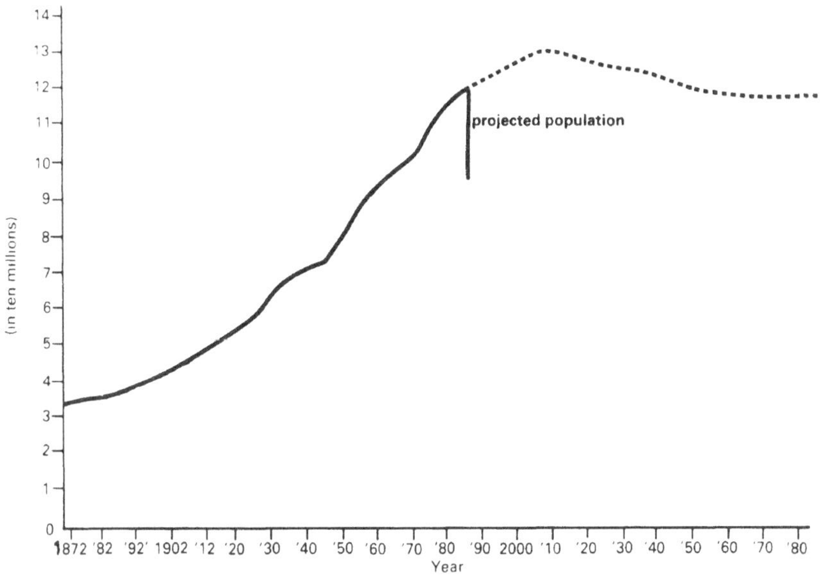

Source: Statistics and Information Department, Ministry of Health and Welfare, Tokyo, 1987

Table 3.2 Population growth and population projections, selected years, 1872–2080

Year	*Population (1,000s)*	*Year*	*Population (1,000s)*
1872	34,806	1986	121,672
1880	36,649	1990	124,225
1890	39,902	2000	131,192
1900	43,847	2010	135,823
1910	49,184	2020	135,304
1920	55,473	2030	134,067
1930	64,450	2040	131,646
1940	71,933	2050	128,681
1950	83,200	2060	126,947
1960	93,419	2070	125,518
1970	103,720	2080	124,401
1980	117,060		

Source: Demographic Statistics, 1986, Institute of Population Problems, Ministry of Health and Welfare, Tokyo, 1986

two decades of the century the birth-rate increased, in contrast to the west where birth-rates were starting to decline. By 1920 the Japanese birth-rate was 36.2 per 1,000 population. In the mid-1920s it started to decline and reached a new low level of 26.6 per 1,000 in 1939. Government propaganda (a need for a strong populous nation) was instrumental in causing an upsurge in the birth-rate during the early part of the war; the return of military and civilian personnel from overseas after the war meant that Japan, just like other countries, experienced a post-war baby boom – 2,578,792 live births in 1947 was the highest number in more than twenty years and shot the birth-rate up to 34.3 per 1,000 population. Between 1950 and 1957 there was a steep drop in the birth-rate. Real per capita income in the years after the war was less than half of pre-war levels and extreme poverty was the prime motive for limiting births. The Eugenic Protection Law of 1948 liberalized abortion and was critical in enabling women to limit births. From 29.1 per 1,000 population in 1950 the birth-rate dropped to 17.2 per 1,000 population in 1960. The years 1960–73 saw a slight increase in the birth-rate as the children born in the early 1940s reached marriage and child-bearing age and Japan experienced its second baby boom. A notable exception to the pattern and one which has an interesting explanation was the year 1966 when there was a steep drop in the number of births (see Figure 3.2).

This was the result of a phenomenon called 'Hi no E Uma' or the

Figure 3.2 Crude birth-rate, Japan, 1920–83

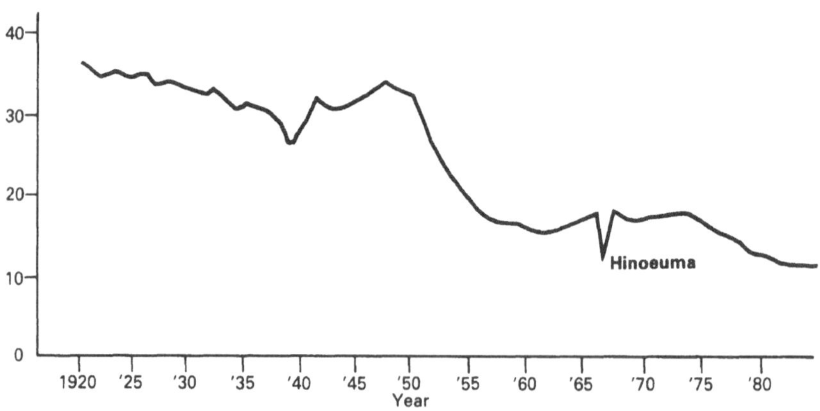

Source: Statistics and Information Department, Ministry of Health and Welfare, Tokyo, 1987

Figure 3.3 Birth-rates, Japan and selected countries, 1900–84

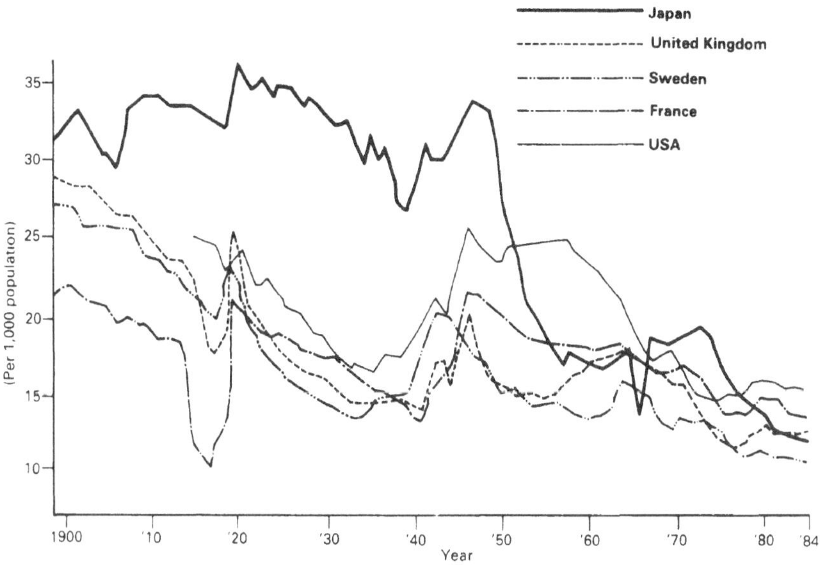

Source: Statistics and Information Department, Ministry of Health and Welfare, Tokyo, 1987

Table 3.3 Crude birth-rates, Japan and selected countries, 1932–84

Year	*Japan*	*UK*	*Sweden*	*France*	*USA*
1932	32.9	15.8	14.5	17.3	17.4
1940	29.4	14.6	15.1	13.6	17.9
1945	—	16.2	20.4	16.2	19.6
1950	28.1	16.3	16.4	20.6	23.5
1955	19.4	15.5	14.8	18.6	24.7
1960	17.2	17.5	13.7	17.9	23.7
1965	18.6	18.3	15.9	17.8	19.4
1966	13.7	17.9	15.8	17.6	18.3
1970	18.8	16.3	13.7	16.7	18.2
1975	17.1	12.5	12.6	14.1	14.6
1980	13.6	13.4	11.7	14.9	15.9
1984	12.5	12.9	11.3	13.8	15.5

Source: UN Demographic Yearbook; *UN Monthly Bulletin of Statistics, 1987*; 'Vital Statistics', Statistics and Information Department, Ministry of Health and Welfare
Note: Japan 1986: 11.4/1,000 population. Ministry of Health and Welfare figures released June 1987.

Year of the Fiery Horse. In addition to naming years after twelve animals the Japanese time system uses the ten celestial stems from Chinese astrology whereby each of the five elements (wood, fire, earth, metal, and water) is divided into two orders, the younger and the elder. The celestial stems and animal signs run concurrently and together produce a 60-year cycle, 60 being the first number divisible by 10 and 12. 'Hi no E' is a fire year with a dominant 'elder' characteristic and 'Uma' is the horse. Old Japanese beliefs have it that women born in the year of the fiery horse are of a troublesome disposition and make very difficult wives. Such women, so some stories go, are even highly likely to consume a man. Modern Japanese undoubtedly do not take such beliefs quite so seriously as their predecessors but none the less prefer not to have children in such a 'difficult' year in order to avoid the risk of having a daughter who might then be difficult to marry off. (Company personnel directors found, at the 1986 round of graduate employment interviews, that there was an uncommonly large number of female applicants born on 30 and 31 December 1965!) A similar drop in the birth-rate was recorded in 1906 and Japanese demographers are keen to see what happens in 2026, the next year of the fiery horse.

Since the 1970s the birth-rate has declined steadily and in 1986 it stood at 11.4 per 1,000 population, the 1,382,976 babies born that year being the second lowest annual number recorded since 1899.[2] We can compare the trend in the Japanese birth-rate with that of other developed countries in Figure 3.3 and Table 3.3.

Death-rates

In 1986 Japan's crude death-rate was 6.2 per 1,000 population, the lowest rate in the world. Age-specific death-rates declined steeply for all age groups from the 1950s onward, but it was the lowering of death-rates in the very youngest age groups (0–4 years and 10–14 years especially) and in the death-rate from tuberculosis in the 1950s which made a particularly important contribution to the overall drop in the death-rate since that time (see Figure 3.4).

The major causes of death in the early Meiji era were acute infectious diseases. Cholera epidemics in 1879 and 1886 were responsible for 105,786 and 108,405 deaths respectively; the estimated population at the time was 36 million and 39 million, therefore some 3 people per 1,000 were dying of the disease. If we compare this with the total death-rate for the country today of 6.2 per 1,000 population, we can fully appreciate why outbreaks of cholera so terrified the community (see Table 3.4).

In the early years of the twentieth century Japan's death-rate

Figure 3.4 Death-rates, Japan and selected countries, 1900–84

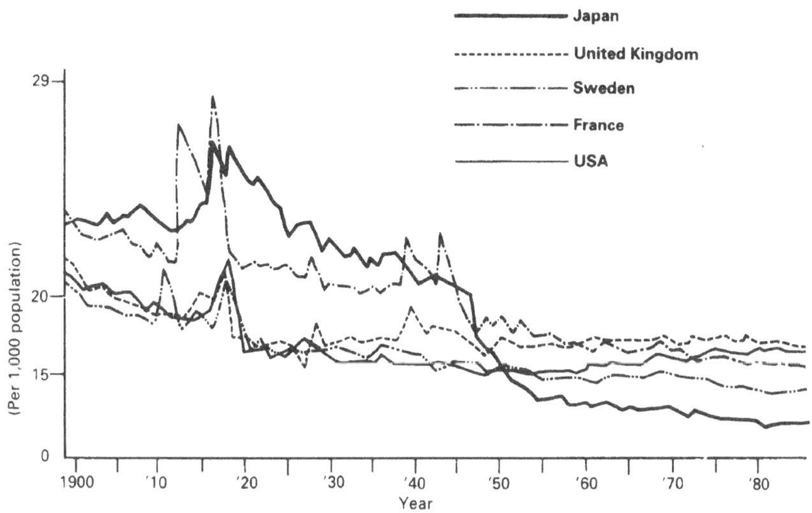

Source: Statistics and Information Department, Ministry of Health and Welfare, Tokyo, 1987

Table 3.4 Deaths from epidemic diseases, 1879–1910

Disease	*1879*	*1880*	*1885*	*1890*	*1895*	*1900*	*1910*
Cholera	105,786	618	9,329	32,227	40,154	—	1,656
Dysentery	1,477	1,305	10,690	8,706	12,959	10,538	9,877
Typhoid fever	2,530	4,177	6,672	8,464	8,401	5,544	8,046
Smallpox	1,295	1,731	3,329	25	268	7	15
Epidemic typhus	601	360	365	67	49	2	1
Diphtheria	534	1,019	1,440	1,438	3,025	6,010	5,415
Plague	—	—	—	—	—	22	237

Source: Statistics on Communicable Diseases, Ministry of Health and Welfare, Tokyo

Table 3.5 Death-rates in the late Meiji era, Japan and selected countries

	Meiji 33 (1900)	*Meiji 38 (1905)*	*Meiji 43 (1910)*
Japan	20.3	21.1	21.1
USA	17.6	16.0	15.0
UK	18.4	15.6	14.0
France	21.9	19.6	17.8
Sweden	16.8	15.6	14.0

Source: UN Demographic Yearbook

remained relatively high when compared with western countries (see Table 3.5) and it did not drop to comparable levels until after the Second World War. Industrial progress and economic growth certainly brought some improvements in the country's living standards in the first two decades of the century but the benefits of progress were distributed unevenly throughout Japanese society. The population grew fast in the rapidly industrializing urban centres, and for a long time housing and working conditions were poor; factories and other work-places were subject to minimum regulations; medical and health services, as we saw in Chapter 2, were developed only sporadically. In the countryside conditions had improved only slightly since the nineteenth century. Modern amenities hardly existed outside the towns and the rural population was still prey to infectious and parasitic diseases. Even as late as the 1950s only one-third of the country was linked to piped water supplies.

The death-rate declined gradually through the 1920s but epidemics of Spanish influenza in 1920 and 1924 meant high death-rates for those years. In the 1930s and 1940s the situation started to improve and death-rates edged closer to those of other modern industrial nations (see Table 3.6). Between 1947 and 1955 the crude death-rate was halved – from 14.6 per 1,000 population it fell to 7.8 per 1,000 population, with the decrease in infant and perinatal mortality accounting for a large portion of the decline. It is worth noting that in the USA and Sweden it took about forty years for the death-rate to decline from 15 per 1,000 population to 10 per 1,000 population. The drop in deaths from infectious diseases – tuberculosis, pneumonia, bronchitis, whooping cough, diphtheria, scarlet fever – was most dramatic. Medical services became more widespread, newly discovered drugs began to be used on a large scale, vaccination programmes were started; nutrition standards were getting better and environmental conditions were changing. Living conditions all round were fast catching up with standards elsewhere in the world.

Japan's very low death-rate at present is attributed primarily to its age structure. As the proportion of elderly people in the population increases, however, as it will do in the next twenty to twenty-five years, the crude death-rate is forecast to rise.

The infant mortality-rate is a sound indicator of socio-economic development and of the general health conditions of a society. In Japan the infant mortality-rate has fallen dramatically over the last forty years. In 1900 more than 150 out of every 1,000 infants born died in the first year of life and such infant deaths accounted for 20 per cent of all deaths in the country. The infant mortality-rate was a high 165.7 per 1,000 live births in 1920, almost double the rates in the UK and the USA. It declined steadily in the 1930s and by

Table 3.6 Death-rates, Japan and selected countries, 1932–84

Year	*Japan*	*UK*	*Sweden*	*France*	*USA*
1932	17.7	12.3	11.6	15.8	10.9
1940	16.5	14.4	11.4	18.5	10.7
1945	—	12.7	10.8	16.6	10.6
1950	10.9	11.7	10.0	12.7	9.6
1955	7.8	11.7	9.5	12.1	9.3
1960	7.6	11.5	10.0	11.4	9.5
1965	7.1	11.6	10.1	11.1	9.4
1970	6.9	11.8	9.9	10.7	9.4
1975	6.3	11.9	10.8	10.6	8.9
1980	6.2	11.7	11.0	10.2	8.7
1984	6.2	11.4	10.9	9.8	8.6

Sources: UN Demographic Yearbook; *UN Monthly Bulletin of Statistics*; 'Vital Statistics', Statistics and Information Department, Ministry of Health and Welfare

Figure 3.5 Infant mortality-rates, Japan and selected countries, 1900–84

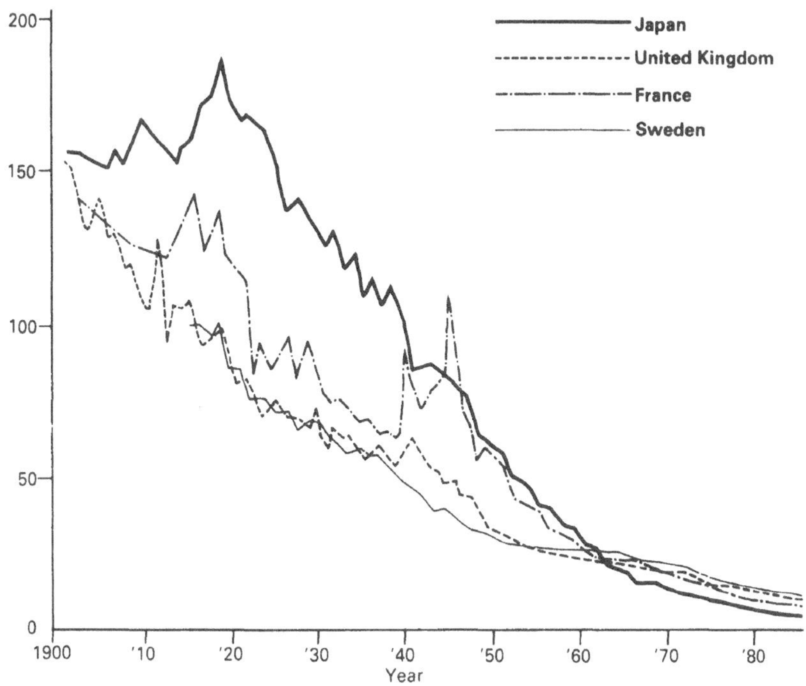

Source: Statistics and Information Department, Ministry of Health and Welfare, Tokyo, 1987

Table 3.7 Infant mortality-rates, Japan and selected countries, 1932–86

Year	*Japan*	*UK*	*France*	*USA*
1932	117.5	68.3	77.0	57.6
1940	90.0	61.0	95.3	47.0
1945	–	48.8	112.7	38.3
1950	60.1	31.4	52.0	29.2
1955	39.8	25.8	38.6	26.4
1960	30.7	22.5	27.4	26.0
1965	18.5	19.6	21.9	24.7
1970	13.1	18.4	18.2	20.0
1975	10.0	16.0	13.8	16.1
1980	7.5	12.1	10.0	12.6
1984	6.0	10.2	9.0[a]	10.6[a]
1986	5.2[b]	–	–	–

Source: UN Demographic Yearbook; 'Vital Statistics', Statistics and Information Department, MHW
Notes: [a]Provisional
[b]Ministry of Health and Welfare figures released June 1987.

1950 was down to 60.1 per 1,000 live births, a substantial improvement but none the less a rate which left Japan a long way behind other developed nations and more on a par with neighbouring Asian countries. As Figure 3.5 shows, the infant mortality-rate fell more rapidly during the 1950s but it is from the early 1960s on that the really massive drop in infant mortality came about as living conditions improved; a comprehensive programme in maternal and child health (MCH) greatly enhanced the care of pregnant women, infants, and young children and was especially important in getting such services out to the rural communities. With her 1986 figure of 5.2 per 1,000 live births Japan has the lowest infant mortality-rate in the world (see Table 3.7).

Turning to average life expectancy at birth we can see that Japan has achieved notable gains since the beginning of the century and most spectacularly in the past forty years. When the first life-table was drawn up at the beginning of the century male life expectancy was 42.8 years and female 44.3 years. Moderate gains were achieved during the first twenty years of the century but the country lagged behind other developed nations. The sixth life-table of 1935/36 showed that a Japanese male could expect to live 46.9 years and a female 49.6 years. Western countries at the time were showing averages closer to 60 years (see Table 3.8).

Greater improvements were made in the immediate post-war years: between 1947 and 1952 life expectancy at birth extended from 50 to 60 years, whereas it had taken some twenty years in the UK and the

Table 3.8 Expectation of life at birth, Japan and selected countries, 1900–80

Year	*Japan*		*UK*[a]		*France*		*USA*	
	M	*F*	*M*	*F*	*M*	*F*	*M*	*F*
1900	43.97	44.85	–	–	45.31	48.69	47.88	50.70
1910	44.25	44.73	51.50	55.35	48.49	52.41	49.86	53.24
1920	—	—	55.62	59.58	52.19	56.09	55.50	57.40
1930	44.82	46.54	58.74	62.88	54.30	59.02	57.71	60.89
1940	50.06	53.96	66.39	71.15	61.87	67.43	64.6	69.9
1950	59.57	62.97	66.49	71.22	63.6	69.3	65.6	71.1
1960	65.32	70.19	68.3	74.1	67.2	73.8	66.6	73.1
1970	69.31	74.66	68.6	74.9	68.6	76.1	67.1	74.8
1980	73.35	78.76	70.4	76.6	70.05	78.20	69.8	77.5

Source: UN Demographic Yearbook; Statistics and Information Department, Ministry of Health and Welfare
Note: [a]England and Wales.

Table 3.9 International comparison of expectation of life at birth

Country	*Year*	*M*	*F*
Japan	1985	74.84	80.46
China	1981	66.43	69.35
India	1975/80	51.20	50.00
Indonesia	1980/85	51.20	53.40
Singapore	1980	68.70	74.00
Canada	1980/82	71.88	78.98
USA	1984	71.1	78.3
Australia	1983	72.09	78.72
New Zealand	1983	70.81	76.92
USSR	1975/80	65.00	74.30
Austria	1983	69.53	76.61
Denmark	1982/83	71.50	77.50
Finland	1983	70.16	77.98
France	1982	70.73	78.85
Germany (DDR)	1983	69.46	75.42
Germany (FDR)	1981/83	70.46	77.09
Iceland	1983/84	73.96	80.20
Italy	1977/79	70.61	77.19
Netherlands	1982/83	72.75	79.48
Norway	1982/83	72.69	79.54
Sweden	1984	73.84	79.89
Switzerland	1982/83	72.80	79.50
England and Wales	1981/83	71.34	77.35

Source: UN Demographic Yearbook

USA to achieve similar gains. By 1985 Japan was leading all other countries, with an average life expectancy of 74.8 years for men and 80.5 years for women (see Table 3.9). According to figures released by the Ministry of Health and Welfare in June 1987 the average life expectancy of both men and women increased by 0.45 years in 1986. The average life expectancy for a newborn male in 1986 was 75.23 years and 80.93 years for a female, keeping Japan in the premier position in the world, with Iceland in second place.

Disease patterns

In Japan, as elsewhere, there have been considerable changes in the incidence and prevalence of certain diseases in the past forty years. The acute infectious diseases which were the major killers in the nineteenth and early twentieth centuries have largely been conquered. In addition to advances in medical sciences and the spread of health care services, improved housing, better nutrition, education, all the components of social and economic development in other words, have worked together to effect these changes in health status. The place of the infectious diseases has been taken by cancer, heart disease, disorders of the cerebral system, the popularly called diseases of civilization. These diseases are not 'new' in Japan just as they are not 'new' in other countries: cerebro-vascular diseases were the third most common cause of death in Japan in 1900 for example. But social and environmental conditions in Japan have changed to such an extent that circumstances now predispose to the greater prevalence of some diseases. Those factors which helped overcome acute infectious diseases, that is the developments in medical science, application of new drugs and therapies have proved less successful at dealing with degenerative diseases. Affluence as much as poverty can have nefarious effects. In Japan affluence has had an added dimension too: 'westernization' has made its own singular contribution to the changing patterns of morbidity and mortality in the country. Japan suffered until relatively later in her socio-economic development from the diseases of poverty and she has, in the past twenty years especially, started to experience the impact of the diseases of affluence. In the following section we shall therefore look more closely at the incidence and prevalence of some diseases noting too some of the similarities or differences between Japan and other countries.

Infectious diseases

Starting with trends in infectious diseases, after the country's surrender in 1945 it was beset by epidemics of infectious diseases – tuberculosis, Japanese encephalitis, poliomyelitis, typhoid, gastroenteritis, whooping cough, diphtheria, scarlet fever. In a country where the majority of the population was severely malnourished, the infrastructure in ruins, and which lacked the most basic medical supplies and equipment, the ideal circumstances existed for the spread of acute infectious diseases in the two years following Japan's surrender. In 1946 for example there were more than 88,000 cases of dysentery (with 13,000-plus deaths), almost 45,000 cases of typhoid fever with more than 5,000 deaths, close to 50,000 cases of diphtheria (and 3,825 deaths) and 17,954 cases of smallpox with just over 3,000 deaths. Between 1947 and 1949 however the occupation forces gradually reorganized medical and health services and implemented sweeping and often compulsory preventive measures (e.g. DDT spraying) and the incidence of many infectious diseases started to drop. Later from the mid-1950s to the mid-1960s there were some serious, large-scale outbreaks of dysentery, typhoid fever, scarlet fever, measles, and influenza but with modern medication and treatment their impact was less severe than in earlier times and the death-rates consequently greatly reduced (see Table 3.10). Of interest is the reappearance of cholera in Japan since the end of the 1970s. Between 1947 and 1976 there were just three notified cases (one in 1963 and two in 1964). In 1977 there were twenty-nine cases and there have been between ten and forty cases per year since then, although a high fifty-five cases were notified in 1984. It is possible that recognition of the disease and hence its reporting by doctors has improved. It is equally likely that there are more cases of cholera because of increased travel abroad for vacation purposes, especially to south-east Asian countries where the disease is still more prevalent, Japanese 'affluence' therefore having its impact.

Tuberculosis, the scourge of factory workers in the early part of the century and the leading cause of death in the 1930s, continued to be so until the beginning of the 1950s. With the Tuberculosis Prevention Act of 1950 the government implemented a subsidized nation-wide screening and prevention programme. Existing in-patient facilities were expanded or improved and new ones set up. The recently developed and potent drugs such as penicillin were used with great effect; as social conditions improved and the general health status of the people rose it was possible to bring the disease under control. In 1950 the tuberculosis death-rate was still high at 146.6 per 100,000 population and it was the leading cause of death that year, but in Japan, as elsewhere, the steady decline of the disease was well under way (see Figure 3.6).

By 1983 the tuberculosis death-rate was down to 4.5 per 100,000

Table 3.10 Numbers of patients and deaths from legal communicable diseases, selected years, 1900–85

Year	*Cholera*		*Dysentery*		*Typhoid fever*		*Diphtheria*		*Smallpox*	
	pts	*deaths*	*pts*	*deaths*	*pts*	*deaths*	*pts*	*deaths*	*pts*	*deaths*
1900	377	–	46,180	10,583	23,846	5,544	17,873	6,010	111	7
1910	2,849	1,656	31,958	9,877	35,378	8,046	19,013	5,415	80	15
1920	14,969	8,417	12,723	8,148	53,756	12,073	15,113	3,801	3,166	729
1930	2	2	29,672	13,041	41,367	8,340	18,522	4,069	7	4
1940	5	5	83,689	22,025	40,706	7,106	38,303	4,728	575	60
1950	—	–	49,780	11,968	4,883	630	12,621	1,182	5	2
1960	—	–	93,971	2,048	1,572	39	14,921	497	–	–
1970	—	–	9,996	51	211	3	596	6	–	–
1980	22	–	951	–	294	1	66	1	–	–
1985	34	–	1,128	6	211	–	10	–	–	–

Source: Statistics on Communicable Diseases, Ministry of Health and Welfare, Tokyo

Figure 3.6 Tuberculosis death-rates, Japan and selected countries, 1910–85

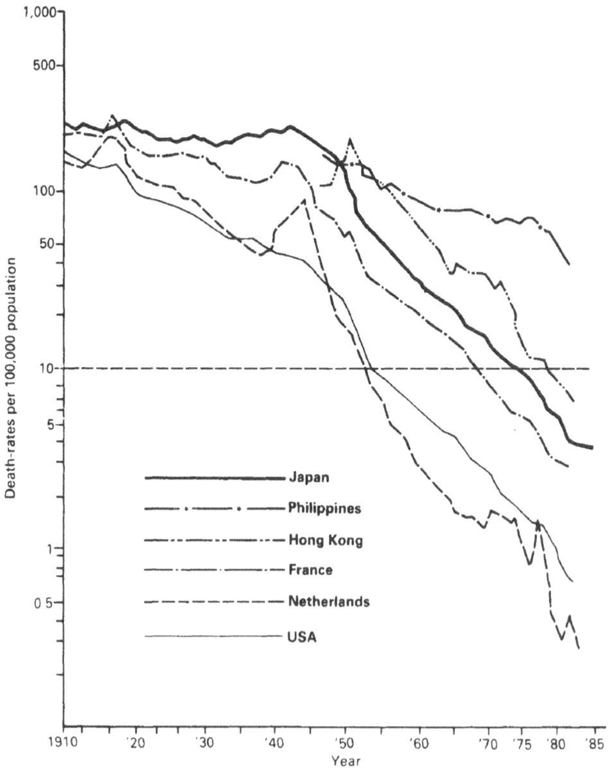

Source: Statistics and Information Department, Ministry of Health and Welfare, Tokyo, 1987

Table 3.11 International comparison of tuberculosis death-rates (per 100,000 population)

Year	*Japan*	*USA*	*England and Wales*	*Italy*	*Denmark*	*France*	*Netherlands*
1947	187.2	33.4	54.7	77.2	30.1	79	37.4
1950	146.4	22.5	36.3	42.6	13.8	57.9	19.0
1955	52.3	9.2	14.6	22.7	6.3	31.3	6.7
1960	34.2	6.1	7.5	17.1	4.2	22.0	2.9
1965	22.8	4.1	4.8	12.9	2.0	14.6	1.8
1966	20.3	3.9	4.9	11.1	1.9	13.3	1.5
1967	17.8	3.5	4.2	9.5	1.7	13.0	1.4
1968	16.8	3.1	4.3	8.9	1.6	10.7	1.5
1969	16.1	2.8	3.8	8.2	2.6	9.9	1.3
1970	15.4	2.7	3.3	7.0	2.8	8.2	1.2
1971	13.0	2.2	2.9	6.8	2.4	7.4	1.5
1972	11.9	2.2	3.0	6.2	2.7	6.9	1.4
1973	11.1	1.8	2.7	5.9	2.6	6.3	1.4
1974	10.4	1.7	2.6	5.0	2.3	6.0	1.3
1975	9.5	1.6	2.6	5.0	1.7	5.5	1.5
1976	8.5	1.4	2.3	4.2	1.9	5.2	1.0
1977	7.8	1.4	2.1	3.7	1.7	4.8	0.7
1978	7.2	1.3	1.8	3.4	1.6	4.6	1.3
1979	5.8	0.9	1.3	3.0	1.7	3.1	0.5
1980	5.5	0.8	1.3	2.7	1.4	3.0	0.3
1981	4.9	0.9	1.2	—	1.6	3.0	0.4
1982	4.5	0.7	1.1	—	0.9	—	0.3

Source: World Health Statistics Annual

population, still higher than the rates in other developed countries (see Table 3.11), but it was responsible for less than 1 per cent of all deaths in the country. Formerly most common among the young it is now found more among the older age groups, as in western countries.

Degenerative diseases

Degenerative diseases have been the leading cause of death in Japan since the 1960s; Table 3.12 illustrates the changes in order of cause of death since the beginning of the century. Cerebral diseases took over from tuberculosis as the leading cause of death in 1951, cancer took second place in 1953, and heart disease moved into third place in 1958. The overall death-rate from cerebro-vascular diseases has been decreasing since the beginning of the 1970s and it dropped into second place in 1981, being replaced by deaths from all cancers. Since 1985 the three major causes of death in Japan, in order, have been cancer, heart disease, and cerebro-vascular diseases, a pattern

Table 3.12 Changes in the order of causes of death

Year/ Order	*No. 1*		*No. 2*		*No. 3*		*No. 4*		*No. 5*	
	Cause of death	*Death-rate per 100,000 population*	*Cause of death*	*Death-rate per 100,000 population*	*Cause of death*	*Death-rate per 100,000 population*	*Cause of death*	*Death-rate per 100,000 population*	*Cause of death*	*Death-rate per 100,000 population*
1900	Pneumonia, bronchitis	226.1	Tuber-culosis	163.7	Cerebro-vascular diseases	159.2	Gastro-enteritis	133.8	Senility	131.0
1910	"	262.0	"	230.2	Gastro-enteritis	213.4	Cerebro-vascular diseases	131.9	"	120.2
1920	"	408.0	Gastro-enteritis	254.2	Tuber-culosis	223.7	Influenza	193.7	Cerebro-vascular diseases	157.6
1930	Gastro-enteritis	221.4	Pneumonia, bronchitis	200.1	"	185.6	Cerebro-vascular diseases	162.8	Senility	118.8
1940	Tuber-culosis	212.9	"	185.8	Cerebro-vascular diseases	177.7	Gastro-enteritis	159.2	"	124.5
1947	"	187.2	"	174.8	Gastro-enteritis	136.8	Cerebro-vascular diseases	129.4	"	100.3
1950	"	146.4	Cerebro-vascular diseases	127.1	Pneumonia, bronchitis	93.2	Gastro-enteritis	82.4	Malignant neoplasms	77.4
1960	Cerebro-vascular diseases	160.7	Malignant neoplasms	100.4	Heart diseases	73.2	Senility	58.0	Pneumonia, bronchitis	49.3

Table 3.12 contd.

Year/ Order	No. 1		No. 2		No. 3		No. 4		No. 5	
	Cause of death	*Death-rate per 100,000 population*	*Cause of death*	*Death-rate per 100,000 population*	*Cause of death*	*Death-rate per 100,000 population*	*Cause of death*	*Death-rate per 100,000 population*	*Cause of death*	*Death-rate per 100,000 population*
1970	Cerebro-vascular diseases	175.8	Malignant neoplasms	116.3	Heart diseases	86.7	Accidents	42.5	Senility	38.1
1980	"	139.5	"	139.1	"	106.2	Pneumonia, bronchitis	33.7	"	27.6
1981	Malignant neoplasms	142.0	Cerebro-vascular diseases	134.3	"	107.5	"	33.7	"	25.5
1982	"	144.2	"	125.0	"	106.7	"	35.0	Accidents	24.7
1983	"	148.3	"	122.8	"	111.3	"	39.3	"	25.0
1984	"	152.5	"	117.2	"	113.9	"	37.6	"	24.6
1985	"	156.1	Heart diseases	117.3	Cerebro-vascular diseases	112.2	"	42.7	"	24.6
1986	"	158.4	"	117.8	"	106.9	"	43.9	"	23.5

Source: 'Vital Statistics', Statistics and Information Department, Ministry of Health and Welfare, Tokyo
Note: Before 1940 and after 1975, Okinawa Prefecture is included.

which differs slightly from most other developed countries. In the United Kingdom, the USA, and Sweden for instance, heart disease ranks first with cancer in second place. In the USA the death-rate from heart disease is declining whereas in the United Kingdom, Sweden, and France the rates for heart-disease-related deaths continue to rise.

Looking specifically at cancer in Japan we can see that the cancer death-rate was relatively low during the first fifty years of the century and it has been estimated that cancer was responsible for 3–5 per cent of all deaths.[3] Cancer deaths began to increase after the Second World War and in 1953 cancer became the second most common cause of death. Since that time both the number of cancer deaths and the crude death-rate from cancer have increased steadily. In 1983 deaths from all types of cancer accounted for 23.8 per cent of all deaths (a cancer death-rate of 148.3 per 100,000 population). By 1986, according to figures released by the Ministry of Health and Welfare in June 1987, cancer deaths made up more than a quarter of all deaths in Japan, 191,602 out of the 750,641 deaths that year.[4] However the percentage of cancer deaths among all deaths varies according to age. Among males in their 50s and 60s cancer was responsible for about 40 per cent of all deaths in 1983; it caused a higher proportion of deaths among women in the same age groups, about 44–45 per cent. Using mortality statistics epidemiologists have calculated that the age-adjusted cancer death-rates in males have none the less remained stable since the 1960s and in females have started to show a decrease since the 1970s. The increased crude cancer death-rate is considered to be a reflection of the changing age structure of the Japanese population, that is it is ageing rapidly, life expectancy has been greatly prolonged, and there is consequently an increased number and proportion of cancer-prone elderly people in the population.[5]

The incidence-rate and death-rate of various site-specific cancers differ slightly in Japan from rates in other countries. On the whole these cancers which are increasing in Japan are those which are the more common in the west and those cancers which are declining in Japan are the cancers which are less common or declined some time ago in western countries. Japan shows differences too in the incidence and death-rate for various cancers according to sex. Stomach cancer accounted for 49,000 or 26 per cent of all cancer deaths in 1985 and was the leading cause of cancer death among men and women alike. It cause 29.6 per cent of all male cancer deaths and 25.7 per cent of all female cancer deaths in 1983.[6]

Lung cancer is the second most common cause of cancer death among males followed by liver cancer, pancreatic cancer, oesophageal cancer and rectal cancer. Lung cancer is likewise the second leading cause of cancer death among women; third is uterine cancer followed by liver cancer, breast cancer, and pancreatic cancer.

The incidence and ranking of various site-specific cancers in Japan is quite different from those found elsewhere. The stomach cancer death-rate puts Japan first among forty-six countries for both males and females.[7] In men the Japanese incidence and death-rates rank relatively high for oesophageal and liver cancer; among women Japan ranks relatively high for the rate of uterine, oesophageal, biliary tract, liver, rectal and lung cancer. Compared to most other countries, however, Japanese women run a very low risk of developing either breast or skin cancer. And for both men and women in Japan the incidence of and death-rates for leukaemia, bone cancer, and thyroid cancer are relatively low. Using data gathered at twelve cancer registries throughout the country together with mortality statistics, Japanese epidemiologists have analysed the trends in cancer incidence, which suggest that the Japanese cancer pattern is changing and in the 1980s is starting to take on the characteristics of western countries.

Stomach cancer Japan still has the highest stomach cancer death-rates in the world but it is significant that the rate of incidence of stomach cancer has been falling over the past twenty-five years and a pattern of decline similar to that seen in the USA in the 1930s is evident in Japan. Japan's higher incidence and mortality from stomach cancer have been attributed primarily to the risk factors associated with the Japanese diet and this has changed greatly over the past forty years. The 'traditional' Japanese diet was high in carbohydrate and low in fat and animal protein; it included a high content of pickled, cured, and fermented ingredients and consumption of these has been identified as increasing the risk of developing stomach cancer. Soy sauce, salt fish, and pickles were and still are eaten in large quantities; historically these ingredients were a necessary way of adding variety and flavour to the staple food, rice. This was particularly so in the rural areas prior to the spread of domestic refrigeration and even more important in the winter months when fresh products were difficult, if not impossible, to obtain. Since the early 1960s Japan's prosperity has enabled people everywhere to acquire the accoutrements of modern living; changes in life-style and the growing popularity of things 'western' and therefore considered modern and fashionable, the development of a highly effective retail marketing and distribution system have all made some contribution to the modification of eating habits.

Excessive salt intake is associated with gastric cancer[8] and hypertension, and it is therefore also a risk factor for cerebrovascular disease. Average daily salt intake per capita in Japan remains high by western standards but it has dropped – from 14.5 gm in 1972 to 12.3 gm in 1982[9] – and there is growing public awareness of the need to cut down salt intake. But what other important changes have taken place in Japan's eating habits? Rice continues as by far and away the leading carbohydrate but consumption of it is in fact declining: its place is being taken by potatoes to some extent, especially in the form of 'french fries' among young people, and more bread is being eaten too. Consumption of milk, butter, margarine, and eggs is increasing. 'Gratin' dishes are popular in restaurants and all supermarkets offer a wide selection of frozen and dried convenience foods of this type. Fresh fish consumption has decreased slightly, matched by an increase in the consumption of all kinds of meat and poultry, although by western standards the size of the portions taken is usually quite small. The 'traditional' breakfast of rice with pickles, broth, and vegetables is rapidly disappearing from many Japanese homes. A large and growing number of families are nowadays far more likely to start the day with a 'typical' breakfast of cereals followed by thick slabs of toasted white bread. Cereals are the same brands as those found the world over, but manufactured locally and generally containing less sugar than European and American versions.

Eating out is one of the leading leisure activities in Japan and the restaurant industry is an enormously profitable, vibrant and varied one. In addition to the great range of restaurants offering the whole gamut of Japanese foods there are now the imports, and fast food chains such as McDonald's (Makudonarudo), Kentucky Fried Chicken, Shakey's Pizza, ice-cream shops, and cookie stalls enjoy enormous popularity and make vast profits. Japan has long had its own 'take-away' foods: 'sushi' shops offer a variety of ready-made combinations which are reasonably priced and therefore save time and effort on the part of the busy housewife.

Technology too has made its contribution to changes in diet and eating habits. Frozen food and dried convenience preparations help cut down the amount of time required to prepare dishes. In the 1980s the microwave oven is proving very popular, not only for reasons of speed and cutting down the time of food preparation, but also as a boon in small cramped Japanese kitchens. Despite the undoubted growth in the popularity of convenience foods the Japanese diet still contains a high proportion of fresh products and they are usually very fresh indeed. In the small kitchen storage space is limited and refrigerators are small and in the country's densely populated cities supermarkets with parking are not the norm. Food shopping is done more frequently in Japan than in the USA or even Europe. Moreover when buying fresh produce the Japanese expect and demand exceptionally high-quality goods. They also expect equally high levels of presentation in food as in other products, that is food must not only be ultrafresh but also look it and be properly presented if it is to sell well. Hygiene regulations are strict and levels of cleanliness in shops and supermarkets are exceptionally high.

Lung cancer After stomach cancer, lung cancer was the second cause of cancer death in both men and women in 1983, with a death-rate of 31.9 and 11.6 per 100,000 respectively. It is particularly disconcerting that the lung cancer death-rate for women has more than doubled since the end of the 1950s. Anyone who has stumbled through the swirling clouds of smoke in any Japanese office or choked their way through a lengthy (and they always are) business meeting will attest to the continuing high rate of smoking in the country: 62.5 per cent of all Japanese men were smokers in 1986,[10] down from 80 per cent in 1960 but none the less high and one of the highest rates in the world. By age group the highest rates are to be found among men in their 20s and 30s, 70 per cent of whom smoked according to a 1986 survey. Among women, 15.5 per cent in their 20s and 13.3 per cent in their 30s were reported as smokers. There are regional differences: Hokkaido has the highest proportion of smokers of both sexes. The Japanese moreover favour extra-strength cigarettes and there are no controls on their tar content. There are no restrictions on cigarette advertising and they are widely promoted on billboards, television, and in the press. The advertisements sell cigarettes and the smoking habit with healthy outdoors images – windsurfing, horse-riding, and skiing figure prominently; or the message says that the smoker is a man in control, he is cool, daring, adventurous and he usually stares meaningfully at the camera. Other advertisements, perhaps the most insidious, are aimed at young people and sell the notion that smoking is 'international' and extremely chic – all the things young informed Japanese aspire to be. Despite the continued onslaught from the tobacco companies cigarette smoking has started to wane, although the drop does not match that which has occurred in Europe and the USA. The government's position on smoking and health is extremely ambiguous. On the one hand there is an official and heavily subsidized cancer prevention programme but associated health education programmes are poorly sponsored and tend, so far, to underplay the risks of smoking in relation to lung cancer and heart diseases. The Japan Salt and Tobacco Monopoly was denationalized in 1985 but the Ministry of Finance still retains a majority shareholding in the replacement company, Japan Tobacco Industry Inc. Furthermore the government has yielded to American pressures in the trade sphere; from April 1987 tariffs on imported US pipe tobacco and cigarettes were abolished, thus making imported cigarettes cheaper in Japan. The anti-smoking lobby feels, quite correctly, that the total market will grow and the number of young and female smokers is likely to increase as a result of this step.[11]

Liver cancer Liver cancer and oesophageal cancer death-rates have decreased in women but in men these death-rates remain high. Liver cancer was the third leading cause of cancer death among males in 1983 (12,604 deaths: 12.1 per cent of all male cancer deaths) and the fourth cause of cancer death among women (5,042: 6.9 per cent of all female cancer deaths).[12] The discrepancy between men and women is thought to be associated with the higher frequency of alcohol consumption among men. In Japan liver cancer often occurs in association with cirrhosis of the liver; the availability of ultrasonography and computerized tomography (CT) scanners has made early diagnosis of liver disease relatively easier, but the disease remains difficult to treat successfully. Health specialists in the country are concerned that mortality rates for both liver cancer and cirrhosis of the liver will stay higher than they need be until more is done to prevent the onset of either disease, something which education programmes and change in habits can achieve.[13]

Breast cancer Another site-specific cancer where the Japanese experience differs from the western one is breast cancer in women. The breast cancer death-rate in 1983 was 7.3 per 100,000 (cf. the USA where it was 22.8 per 100,000 in 1981). Diet rather than genetics or race is thought to be a vital factor; the explanation seems to be that the traditional low-fat Japanese diet has conferred substantial protection against the disease. Japanese women living in the USA have the same incidence rate for the disease as Americans and it will be interesting to see if incidence of the disease will be higher among the women who have grown up eating a more westernized diet than their mothers.

The principal reasons for the changes in cancer death-rates in Japan are thought to be changes in the incidence of various cancers the prime influences on which have been life-style and other environmental risk factors. Key among these are diet (the relative proportions of different types of food in the diet and for men drinking habits) and smoking, factors over which individuals have a certain amount of control. Environmental factors include indoor pollution, air pollution, and stress, which is a common aspect of everyday living in Japan's overcrowded cities. There have been changes too in such things as physical activity; children nowadays watch television when they used perhaps to have played; modern amenities reduce the amount of physical labour required to accomplish household and other tasks. Even rice-growing is highly mechanized and requires much less manual labour than twenty years ago. As in the west the Japanese have gradually become far more sedentary.

Cancer screening programmes and improvements in diagnostic and therapeutic techniques may have had a small role to play in the decreases in stomach and uterine cancer death-rates. The government's cancer control programme started in 1965 and offers mass screening for stomach and cervical cancers. The exact numbers reached by the programmes are hard to quantify but the total numbers participating in screening or taking the opportunity for regular check-ups are a very small proportion of the population. For example 3.8 million people underwent some form of cancer screening in 1980 – a large number but a small part of the 117 million-plus population. Official efforts to control cancer have focused for the most part on such screening programmes but more efforts are needed to improve health education programmes and other activities which might help to prevent cancer. First and foremost much more needs to be done in Japan to improve public knowledge about the role of cigarette smoking in relation to lung cancer and heart disease; official attitudes are certainly somewhat cavalier and until these change any efforts to reduce smoking will remain flabby. Japanese epidemiologists have estimated that lung cancer will become the commonest form of the disease in the country by the end of the century and that the lung cancer death-rate will exceed the stomach cancer death-rate as early as 1992 in men and 1997 in women.[14] This is certainly one area where Japan should not wish to emulate the west. Cancer of the colon, breast, and biliary tract are also predicted to increase, thanks to changes in diet and life-style. The incidence and death-rate for stomach cancer will continue to decrease but it will still be relatively more common in Japan than elsewhere for the near future.

Cerebro-vascular and heart diseases Cerebro-vascular disease mortality has been higher in Japan than in other industrial nations throughout the century. Cerebro-vascular disease was the leading cause of death in the country between 1951 and 1980; it fell into second place between 1981 and 1985 when it was superseded by deaths from heart disease (see Table 3.12). In 1983 it was the leading cause of death among women (74,249: 21.9 per cent of all female deaths that year) and second in men (71,631: 17.8 per cent of all male deaths).

Deaths from heart disease ranked third from 1960 until 1985 when it moved into second place. The death-rate from heart disease grew considerably from 1960 when it was 73.2 per 100,000 population to 1984 when it was 113.9 per 100,000 population. As with the incidence of stomach cancer changes in risk factors associated with diet and life-style are considered to have been the major reason why the patterns of heart disease and cerebro-vascular disease have changed. 'Westernization' of the Japanese diet is considered to be responsible for the replacement of cerebro-vascular disease by heart disease. Excessive salt intake is closely related to the development of hypertension and, as we saw in the discussion of cancer, average daily salt intake in Japan is high, even though it is presently decreasing. The decline in salt intake, in addition to contributing to the decline in the incidence of stomach cancer, is thought to have been important in helping reduce the incidence of cerebro-vascular disease. Japanese epidemiologists have compared the relationship between intake of thirty food items and mortality from cerebro-vascular disease and their conclusions have suggested that there were statistically significant correlations for several food items. Rice, starchy roots, miso (soybean paste), pickled vegetables, pork, salted fish, and algae (seaweed) were all positively associated with cerebro-vascular disease.[15]

The intake of meat, fish, milk, and other dairy products increased from the 1960s and as a result the proportion of lipid and protein intakes, especially the proportion of animal protein out of total protein, increased. Carbohydrate intake decreased. The same study found that wheat, butter, margarine, eggs, and beef were negatively associated with cerebro-vascular mortality. In areas of the country where changes in diet have been slower to take place (the north-east, remote country areas, for example) it has been the case that cerebro-vascular mortality has continued to remain high. While a degree of westernization of the diet is therefore positive in that it may contribute to decreasing cerebro-vascular disease there is at the same time the danger that too excessive a change in Japan's eating habits will expose the Japanese to increased risks of heart disease. A balanced approach therefore seems desirable for the prevention of either disease. Other risk factors for heart disease include the inevitable stresses of life in a modern, dynamic, and densely populated society. The increasing employment of women will mean a growing reliance on convenience foods and will therefore be an important factor in dietary changes.

Suicide

It is noteworthy that in 1986 25,659 people committed suicide in Japan, the highest figure ever recorded. Suicide is the leading cause of death in men aged 25–39, but suicide by men in their 40s and 50s is also high. A study by the National Police Agency of suicides in 1985 suggested that despair over illness was the prime motive in more than 40 per cent of suicides. Among executives, concern over work was responsible for about a quarter of all suicides. In 1985 eighty-three children aged under 14 committed suicide: in more than 40 per cent of these cases difficulty at school was the prime motive. The Japanese health care system, as we shall learn, is structured to deal primarily with physical symptoms and poorly equipped to serve the needs of those who might require help with other kinds of problems.

Pollution-related diseases

The Japanese word 'kogai' literally means public injury and is often used in a broader sense than the English term 'environmental pollution'. In this section we shall look at some of the 'kogaibyo' or pollution-related diseases which are found in Japan and which fall into roughly three broad categories – air pollution cases, water pollution cases, and land pollution cases. The enactment of the Pollution Countermeasures Basic Law in 1967 marked the beginning of serious efforts at pollution control and regulation in Japan. The single-minded pursuit of industrial growth in the 1950s and 1960s had taken place without any serious regard for the impact of industrial activity on the environment. After specific outbreaks of diseases which were found to be related to pollution, groups of victims sought legal recourse (always a last and desperate step in a non-litigious society) in the mid-1960s because of the refusal of various industrial concerns to acknowledge any responsibility and because of inaction on the part of government. The ensuing court cases established important legal principles regarding responsibility and liability for injuries to health; they focused public attention on the plight of the victims; raised public consciousness about the need to protect the environment in the interests of the community's health.

We shall look first at air pollution. In industrial areas of Japan such as Yokohama, Kawasaki, Yokkaichi, and Amagasaki in the 1950s and early 1960s the frequency of respiratory disorders such as chronic cough, asthmatic attacks, bronchitis, and pulmonary emphysema increased. Sulphur oxides and nitrogen oxides released into the atmosphere by the combustion of organic materials are known to be the principal causal agents of such disorders. A large proportion of Japan's oil imports comes from the Middle East and such oil contains an average of 2.5 per cent sulphur and releases sulphur oxides more readily than oil from other sources. The prevalence of respiratory disorders was highest in the localities mentioned above, where large quantities of oil were burned in chemical plants. In 1966 atmospheric concentration of sulphur oxides was highest – 0.057 ppm. With the enactment of measures such as the desulphurization of fuel oil and exhaust smoke and other stricter environmental measures the figure was reduced to 0.02 ppm by the end of the 1970s. Respiratory disorders may have other causes such as smoking and it is necessary to have epidemiological evidence and support to establish the exact cause of such diseases. But there are now twenty-three designated air-pollution areas in Japan (including Tokyo, Yokohama, Osaka, and Nagoya) and public health authorities are required to monitor the number of cases of respiratory disorders. In 1975 there were 19,281 officially designated patients; in 1984 89,053 such patients.

Water pollution has provided the most dramatic and horrifying example of environmentally caused disease, Minamata disease being the most notorious. An epidemic outbreak of a disease similar to poliomyelitis occurred in Kumamoto Prefecture on the southern island of Kyushu between 1953 and 1960, with a peak in the number of cases in 1956. As most of the cases were in Minamata City the syndrome was called Minamata disease. It has since become synonymous for the worst of humanity's disregard for the environment. By 1971 there had been 121 confirmed cases, which included 47 dead and 22 cases of congenital Minamata disease observed in newborn infants. Minamata disease remains a matter of controversy and debate as legal requirements for official designation as a sufferer of the disease (and hence for compensation) are still not fully resolved. As of 1981 there were more than 8,000 applicants for medical verification of Minamata disease in Kumamato Prefecture; less than half of those people had completed the process. That the application is not always successful may be seen in more recent figures. In 1984 2,578 people were officially verified as Minamata disease patients and were legally entitled to compensation. Of those verified 656 (25.4 per cent) have died.[16] Full and accurate diagnosis of the disease remains problematic and this has hindered the legal process of obtaining compensation by the victims.[17]

Symptoms of Minamata disease include numbness of the extremities, loss of hearing, clumsiness in small movements, impaired gait and speech, tremor and ataxia. Mental disorders occur in serious cases and children who have congenital Minamata disease are prone to mental retardation. Most victims of Minamata disease were fishermen and their families but symptoms were observed in the local cat and crow population. Researchers at the Faculty of Medicine at Kumamoto University played an important role in plotting and eventually confirming the cause of the disease. Having extracted methyl-mercury compound crystals from a Minamata chemical plant's effluent the blame was fixed on organo-mercury compounds. Total mercury concentration was measured; the mercury concentrate in the fish and shellfish population of Minamata Bay was 10 ppm, 2.5 ppm was present in the brains of patients, 281–760 ppm in their hair: 6 ppm is a normal expected reading.

The pollutant chain was eventually plotted and established: water pollution from the acetaldehyde synthesizing plant of Chisso Corporation in Minamata City marked the beginning of the chain. The process of acetaldehyde synthesization involved introducing acetylene into dilute sulphuric acid, which contained mercuric sulphate as a catalyst; methyl mercury compounds were formed as a by-product of the process. Since at the time knowledge about the process and the end-results was incomplete untreated liquid waste was discharged directly into Minamata Bay. Investigation established that the total concentration of mercury in the bottom of Minamata Bay averaged 50 ppm near the plant, and 2,000 ppm at the drainage outlet itself. The growth in the number of patients paralleled the sharp increase in the production of acetaldehyde at the plant. The mercury was transmitted to the animal and human population of the area via the fish in the bay. Once the pollutant chain was confirmed fishing was, and remains today, prohibited. The matter of compensation for the victims was a long-drawn-out battle in the courts but Chisso finally lost its case and was charged with making compensatory payments to victims. The company did however receive national and prefectural government loans to enable it to do so.

A second outbreak of a disease similar to Minamata disease occurred in the mid-1960s in another fishing and farming district, this time in Niigata Prefecture. The number of cases eventually reached about 1,000 and included 73 deaths. Both the symptoms and pathology of the disease were similar to Minamata disease and mercury was again discovered to be responsible. High levels of mercury were found in the hair of sufferers and others who ate a good deal of fish, in this instance a freshwater river fish. Again a chemical company, the Showa Denko Company and specifically its Kanose plant, was found to have discharged untreated waste and by-products of the acetaldehyde synthesizing process and eventually found to be liable for injury. Legal action was initiated in 1967 and a settlement was reached, with the company's agreeing to compensate victims at rates similar to those agreed for Minamata victims. It is perhaps ironic that advances in petrochemistry have now rendered the acetaldehyde synthesizing process obsolete and no such plants now operate in Japan. Medical science and knowledge on the other hand cannot do anything to cure the victims of these industrial accidents. Only care and comfort can be offered; in a country where conformity to the accepted norm is of tremendous importance, the innocent victims of these diseases still encounter indifference and discrimination. Financial compensation has been slow in coming and does not always cover the provisions for health and other forms of care which may be required. In Kumamoto staff of the National Institute for Minamata Disease carry out a wide range of research programmes, monitoring the sufferers of the disease, and have mounted long-term follow-up studies of the survival rates and incidence of other diseases among the Minamata victims. A welfare centre has been set up so that victims and their families can meet to receive medical treatment and counselling, and a sheltered workshop enables them to receive education and training.

It is clear that there have been considerable changes in the patterns of death and the incidence and prevalence of many diseases in Japan: the changes are leading to increased demand for health and medical care. But the services required from the 1980s are not simply clinical but should be a mix of social welfare and health care programmes if they are to meet adequately the needs of the Japanese people. How the country is tackling the new realities in health care forms the basis of our presentation of information about the Japanese health care system in the following chapters.

References

1 T. Kuroda, 'The demographic transition in Japan', *Social Science and Medicine*, 12A, 451–7, 1978.
2 *Daily Yomiuri*, 25 June 1978.
3 S. Tominaga, 'Cancer trends in Japan from the viewpoint of epidemiology', *Asian Medical Journal*, 29, 1, 35–45, 1986.
4 *Daily Yomiuri*, 25 June 1987.
5 Tominaga, 'Cancer trends in Japan'.
6 *Health and Welfare Statistics in Japan, 1985*, Tokyo, Health and Welfare Statistics Association, 1985, pp. 52–3.
7 Tominaga, 'Cancer trends in Japan'.
8 Y. Ohno, 'Health development in Japan: determinants, implications and perspectives', *WHO Statistics Quarterly*, 38, 2, 176–92, 1985.
9 Ibid.
10 *Japan Times*, 27 January 1987.
11 B. Watanabe, 'Lung cancer: the new import', *Japan Times*, 19 October 1986.

12 *Health and Welfare Statistics in Japan*, 1985.
13 S. Tonuchi, 'Correlation of liver cirrhosis and primary liver cancer in Japanese rural areas', *Japan=Hospitals*, 6, 65–72, July 1987.
14 Tominaga, 'Cancer trends in Japan'.
15 T. Ohmura, S. Hisamatsu, Y. Takizawa, M. Minowa, H. Yanagawa, and I. Shigematsu, 'Geographical distribution of cerebro-vascular disease mortality and food intake in Japan', *Social Science and Medicine*, 24, 5, 401–7, 1987.
16 H. Tamashiro, M. Arakaki, H. Akagi, M. Futukatsu, and Lewis H. Roht, 'Mortality and survival for Minamata disease', *International Journal of Epidemiology*, 14, 4, 582–8, 1985.
17 K. Sonoda, 'SMON and other socially induced diseases in Japan', *Social Science and Medicine*, 12A, 497–506, 1978.

Chapter four

Government policies and provisions for health care

Our purpose in Chapters 4–6 is to provide an up-to-date account of the structure and functions of the principal components of health and medical services in Japan today. We shall be looking therefore at official government policies for the organization and delivery of health and medical services; at mechanisms for the financing of public health services and personal medical care; at the system of medical benefits and contributions, reimbursements to the service-providers and cost-sharing; and lastly at the organization of hospital services and ambulatory care.

But first in Chapter 4 we shall look in detail at government involvement in health care in Japan; at the substance of official policies for the health and medical services, how these have evolved, and the underlying influences affecting official decisions. We shall attempt to describe the nature of and the principal actors in the policy-making process, the central policy-making machinery, and as far as it is possible to do so illustrate with specific examples the usual processes whereby policies are implemented.

Health care policy

We pointed out in Chapter 1 that any country's health care services evolve as an integral part of its political, economic, and administrative infrastructure; they are a reflection and an indicator of its history and present socio-cultural environment and are shaped by its cultural and social traditions. In order to understand fully the nature of policy development for health care and the policy-making process which comes into play in the implementation of health and medical services in Japan today some understanding of the country's political history and present political structure is vital.

Modern Japan: the political background

Japan is an island country with an almost ethnically uniform population, speaking one language and enjoying a common culture. For some 200 years until the middle of the nineteenth century the agrarian, feudal society under the rule of the Tokugawa Shogunate experienced almost total isolation from the rest of the world. With the Meiji Restoration Japan emerged from her cocoon, went on to become the first fully modernized industrial nation in Asia, and within one hundred years became the world's third most powerful economy. In this period of time, just over one hundred years, Japan's political structure has undergone two major changes as a result of external influences. In Chapter 2 we saw how the government set about clearing away the antiquated social and administrative systems of the Tokugawa regime and embarked on a well-planned and thoroughly pragmatic programme of reform and modernization. Administrative and political reforms were undertaken to create a stable and clearly defined government. The political leadership of the day considered that in the advanced countries of the west, constitutions and regulated instruments of government were key elements in their strength, stability, and success; and so Japan should have one too. Ito Hirobumi (1841–1909), one of the country's elder statesmen, visited numerous European countries to study their constitutions and ascertain which kind would be most suitable for adoption, refinement, and assimilation. He was instrumental in drawing up Japan's new constitution which was formally promulgated by the Emperor in 1889.[1]

The new political system thus introduced was highly centralized and authoritarian. Power was concentrated in the hands of a small and elite group who were the Emperor's advisers. Ministers were responsible to the Emperor and his advisers rather than to the two-house Parliament, the Diet. The Lower House – the House of Representatives – was a fully elected body although the electorate was greatly circumscribed, consisting as it did only of those men who paid 15 yen a year in taxes. The Upper House – the House of Peers – comprised former feudal lords, imperial nominees, and a few representatives of the larger taxpayers: it is similar to the House of Lords in the British Parliament, but it could exercise greater authority if it wished to do so. The Constitution also delineated the rights and duties of all citizens – quite a novelty for a country barely out of feudalism. The Meiji Constitution was an important step in bringing democratic processes and principles into Japanese political life, although popular participation in the political process was limited and not even especially sought-after.

Japan's political leaders were astute enough to perceive what we might call the 'public relations' value of a Constitution *per se*; it elevated the country to the ranks of the 'civilized' nations and the Japanese could henceforth consider themselves to be bona fide members of this elite group.

Japan continued to make great strides industrially and economically and by 1912 when Emperor Meiji died the country had achieved recognition as an industrial and military power of some stature. Certainly earlier fears of being overrun by the more powerful and advanced western nations appeared groundless as Japan became confident enough to emulate other imperial powers, and embarked on colonial exploits of her own, taking Korea and Formosa (later Taiwan) as her first imperial possessions. Military strength was seen to bring with it not only independence but also international respect and power.

The essential weaknesses of the Meiji Constitution, together with the prevailing strength of traditional social customs underlying the gloss of modernity, proved critical in shaping Japan's political progress during the 1920s and 1930s as the country industrialized on a massive scale and consolidated her steady economic progress.

The Imperial Household and the Privy Council exercised a great deal of power; the Bureaucracy and the Chiefs of Staff of the Armed Forces all had access to and could advise the Emperor independently of the Cabinet and they exercised this right to the full. The elder statesmen who had been involved in the Restoration of 1868 held the system together by advising the Emperor on various matters, including crucially the selection of suitable candidates for Prime Minister. But by the 1920s these influential, respected and on the whole moderate leaders had either died or withdrawn from public life and they were not replaced by individuals of such outstanding character or ability. There were frequent changes of Prime Minister and Cabinet members; Japanese politics in the 1920s was turbulent as rival factions constantly jockeyed for power. Politicians were universally distrusted as being corrupt and allowing the interests of the giant industrial and financial conglomerates, the 'zaibatsu', to dominate political affairs. The Japanese public did not actively participate in political affairs.

Effective authority gradually fell into other hands, notably those of the military which, like the people, distrusted political party government. The Japanese themselves call the 1930s the 'kurai tanima' (the dark valley), a time of rising ultranationalism, unchecked military aggression abroad, economic troubles, and political suppression of opposition forces at home. The civilian government was constantly thwarted in its aims by younger army officers who resorted to outright disobedience and finally assassination. The army's independence and autonomy of action were enhanced by the requirement that the ministers of the army and navy had to be active serving officers, and without the military ministers the Cabinet could not be formed; by the appropriate threats the military could therefore force the Cabinet to do its will. Not only was the executive weak but also it was not always clear who in fact the executive was supposed to be. The opposition was flabby, represented by academics and intellectuals who in popular terms were untrustworthy because they were held to represent foreign ideas. For

> the conflict between modern and traditional was also a conflict between alien and Japanese, arousing once again the emotions of the Meiji struggles. Accordingly Conservatism was argued not only in terms of political antiquarianism, but also in those of 'national essences' and cultural purity.[2]

By the 1930s Japan presented an unpalatable spectacle to the rest of the world. The civilian government was powerless to control an army which launched aggression in Manchuria in 1931, conducted terrorist attacks in Tokyo, holding the whole city at bay for several days in 1932, and eventually as a result of its exploits in Manchuria caused the withdrawal of the country from the League of Nations in 1933. The first phase of Japan's modern history ended in a war which brought not only defeat but also the seeming total destruction of everything the country had achieved since the Meiji Restoration. At the end of the Second World War Japan had to 'bear the unbearable' of surrender and occupation by a foreign power. The American Occupation lasted almost seven years and was a remarkable experience for both sides involved.

Occupation policy was divided into three phases: first came demilitarization, next reform and democratization, and finally economic rehabilitation. The American Occupation Authorities under the leadership of General MacArthur wrote a new constitution for Japan in 1946, which was put into effect in May 1947 and introduced deep, basic changes in Japan's whole political and social structure. The underlying goal of the Americans was to sweep away those aspects of the Meiji Constitution which were considered dangerous and undemocratic. The post-war political system that was shaped by the American Occupation was grounded in extended political participation and clarification of responsibility. At the same time political traditions could not be ignored and have in fact subsequently imposed their own characteristics on the actual workings of the political process in the past forty years.

The Constitution of 1947 clarified the position of the Emperor as 'the symbol of the State and of the unity of the people'. A parliamentary system similar to that in Britain was established; the Diet is the 'highest organ of state power' and the 'sole law-making authority of the state' (Article 41). The two chambers – the Lower Chamber or House of Representatives and the Upper Chamber or House of Councillors – are elected, although the terms of office of Representatives differ. Executive power is vested in the Cabinet headed by the Prime Minister, who like other ministers must be a civilian; the Cabinet is collectively responsible to the Diet (Article 66). The House of Representatives chooses the Prime Minister, who is free to choose his ministers with the proviso that the majority are Diet members. It is rare that this is not the case and in practice the Prime Minister's freedom of choice is restricted only, but critically, by internal party politics. The Constitution also spelled out the human rights of the people, including female suffrage; it is of course famous for Article 9, Japan's explicit renunciation of war as an instrument of foreign policy. Other major reforms achieved by the Occupation were land reform; anti-monopoly legislation broke up the great 'zaibatsu' and aimed at decentralizing the economy, and reform of the education system opened up higher education to a greater proportion of the population.

Since the early 1950s politics in Japan have been characterized by definite trends towards centralization; an important factor in the consolidation of central government power has been the dominant position of the Liberal Democratic Party (LDP), which has been the ruling party since 1955. LDP dominance for so long has enabled the establishment of a formidable political and administrative machine, which includes government ministries and the nation's most powerful interest groups in business, industry, and agriculture. It has helped it to push through certain policies and programmes (those conducive to economic growth) and to hold back on welfare and other programmes because it can resist almost any kind of political opposition and especially that which might, as elsewhere, come from opposition parties, trade unions, or other interest groups.

The concentration of power achieved by the LDP is at the same time limited by a distinctive feature of the Japanese political system, factionalism. All political parties are made up of different factions, which are often in effect mini-parties. For the opposition factionalism has been counter-productive as it has crippled efforts to develop a cohesive party policy with which to fight the ruling party effectively. Within the LDP itself the factions largely concern themselves with wheeling and dealing of favours such as Cabinet positions, the distribution of funds, and organizing of party presidential elections. The Prime Minister often has to shuffle the Cabinet simply because it is the turn of another faction within the party to have a particular portfolio. These kinds of changes often strike the observer as being unnecessary but they do accord with Japanese culture and the requirement that unity and cohesiveness of the group take precedence over individual achievement.

One result of the constant swapping of ministers is that they can exercise only very weak control over their ministries and cannot put their individual stamp on policy even to the same extent that say a British Cabinet minister can. The power of civil servants is consequently much enhanced in the Japanese system. Again because the LDP has been in an unchallenged position for so long communications between the party and the ministries and other important pressure groups are exceptionally good: a commonality of interests is readily achieved. The Japanese political system is therefore one in which power is shared by a limited number of institutions which are characterized by seemingly contradictory features of stability, consensus, and differences of goals.

Health policy: the historical framework

We can distinguish several distinct phases in the evolution of modern health care policy in Japan. The first phase commenced with the Meiji Restoration and lasted until Japan's defeat in 1945. During the early part of this phase government policy was clear-cut – modernization of medical education and practice was paramount and we described this in detail in Chapter 2. Government focus was on the development of medical education; it coincidentally fostered the development of western-style hospitals as the facilities affiliated with the Imperial Medical Schools grew into centres of excellence, enjoying both popular and professional esteem as they do today. The political strength of the medical profession was established in this phase and the medical profession, via the Japan Medical Association, continues to exert a profound influence on government health care policy in the closing years of the twentieth century.

One notable feature of the German medical system which the government did not immediately adopt was health or social insurance to help individuals pay for medical treatment. The government of the day essentially undertook the modernization of medical care because it considered it to be an important feature of a modern industrial nation; any benefits to individuals, while welcome, were not the major preoccupation. So government policy did not extend to the formulation of plans for the organization of services and the provision for personal medical care became the province of entrepreneurial private practitioners, who were at liberty to charge whatever they wanted for their services. When government did eventually turn its attention to health care financing it was motivated not by any humanitarian concerns, but by worries that deterioration in the overall health status of the labour force would have a deleterious effect on Japanese industry and might thus impede Japan's chances of becoming one of the world's leading military and industrial powers.

The government slowly assumed responsibility for public health matters but did not engage in anything like the same level and scale of public health work such as the development of infrastructure, clean water supplies, and sewerage systems as did the public health reformers of England in the nineteenth century. Indeed in the rapidly growing Japanese cities much of this work was left to the increasingly powerful 'zaibatsu' who needed the infrastructure to ensure the efficient working of their factories. Their work in this regard thus set a pattern for the future. In rural areas local communities voluntarily organized associations and community action groups to monitor standards of hygiene and public health and to carry out education and other programmes. Village hygiene associations, mostly run by housewives, were widespread in the countryside and their activities filled in the gaps of non-existent government programmes.

In line with the prevailing paternalistic management practices of the early twentieth century some of the larger industrial groups had begun to provide clinics and health services for their employees and a few had set up voluntary insurance or mutual aid societies. In order to improve a poor situation the government enacted the first piece of social welfare legislation in the country's history and indeed the first of its kind in any Asian country, a fact of which the Japanese were singularly proud. This was the Health Insurance Law of 1922, enacted in 1927, the delay being caused to some extent by the Great Kanto Earthquake of 1923 and its aftermath.

Health insurance was available for employees in factories with fifteen or more workers: they received benefits in the form of medical treatment and cash payments for sickness and occupational injuries. Dependants were not included and the total numbers enrolled initially were estimated at fewer than 2 million; the total population at the time was close to 56 million.[3] No cover was provided for self-employed, agricultural, and domestic workers nor for those working in small family businesses. Militaristic concerns and the need for conciliatory gestures directed at appeasing labour unrest again prompted government action in the late 1930s to extend social and health insurance schemes. The Health Insurance Law of 1938 introduced sickness insurance for farming and fishing communities – still the largest proportion of the population despite rapid industrialization and urbanization. Some benefits for dependants were included in the early 1940s. The pattern established in the first phase was one of incremental and uneven development, which has been the hallmark of the whole social insurance system in Japan and remains so today.

The revolutionary democratic political system introduced by the Occupation marked the start of the next major phase in Japanese health policy; it went in tandem with the country's recovery in the 1950s, continued through the economic resurgence of the 1960s, and finished with the end of the 1970s. The Constitution of 1947 provided the legal framework and philosophical impetus for social security policy until the 1970s. The Constitution guarantees the people's right to life and establishes state responsibility to promote and improve welfare, social security, and public health. Article 25 states:

> All people shall have the right to maintain the minimum standards of wholesome and cultural living. In all spheres of life the state shall use its endeavours for the promotion and extension of social welfare and security and of public health.

This emphasis on human rights and state responsibility for public health and welfare promulgated and legally enshrined a radical development in Japanese society; it also suggested a massive reversal of both popular and official traditional attitudes and values. These new-found values probably reflected more accurately the thinking and ideals of the Constitution's American drafters than those of the Japanese recipients who would have to make a substantial turn-about in thinking about the state's role in health and welfare if the goals of the Constitution were to be fulfilled. However, Japanese politicians were mindful of the upheaval and disorder of the 1930s and so embarked with some enthusiasm on a new course for the country.

In the 1950s the country was still trying to haul herself back on her feet and ideas about comprehensive welfare policies took a back seat while the authorities got on with the more pressing task of economic recovery. Living conditions after the war were appalling and the standard health indices show a nation now at least some fifty years behind those countries she had sought so eagerly to equal and surpass back in the 1920s and 1930s. In 1947 the infant mortality-rate was 76.7 per 1,000 live births; the maternal mortality-rate was almost twice that of the United Kingdom and the USA. In the same year the leading causes of death were tuberculosis, pneumonia and bronchitis, gastro-enteritis and cerebro-vascular disease. In these trying times government priorities for health were necessarily straightforward and practical; they were to get basic medical services back in operation, control and eradicate infectious diseases, and improve maternal and child health (MCH) standards. With the TB Prevention Act of 1950 the government launched a massive nation-wide programme to eradicate the disease. The whole population underwent TB screening; the cost of this and any subsequent treatment was met by the government.

In 1950 there were 467 specialist TB sanatoria, more than half of which were either national or local government facilities; TB beds constituted a quarter of all available hospital beds at the time. In the same year there were also one hundred special communicable diseases facilities, all but four of which were government sponsored. Facilities for the care and treatment of TB patients made up a large proportion of all health facilities right up to the 1960s, and accounted for a major share of government health expenditure. Thanks to the massive input of funds, official commitment, and the determined implementation of programmes, control of TB was achieved and by 1970 it had dropped to ninth place in the overall causes of death in Japan. By 1960 too the infant mortality-rate had fallen to 30.7 per 1,000 live births. Growing economic prosperity and commensurate improvements in living conditions together with the implementation of nation-wide MCH programmes in the mid-1960s resulted in a further drop in the infant mortality-rate.

Policy-makers and health care specialists could now turn their attention to two pressing health care issues: first, the development of a nation-wide, uniformly distributed network of medical care facilities, and second, the implementation of suitable systems of financing medical and health care. The goal of public policy for health was to ensure equity and easy access to an acceptable quality of health and medical care for the whole population.

Let us look first at what happened regarding facilities development. The New Medical Service Law of 1948 superseded previous legislation and established the legal basis and definitions for the development and regulation of health care facilities such as hospitals and clinics. There was an opportunity for a total reorganization of the existing 'system' of health care in Japan at this time (indeed the Occupation forces had recommended this) but the nature of the system itself, together with the long-established political power of its leading exponents, the doctors, ensured that the essential elements of pre-war provisions were not fundamentally altered. The Medical Care Council set up to review health and medical provisions and to plan for future developments was particularly concerned about the maldistribution of physicians and hospitals within the country: many rural areas were still without any provision for medical care. It was unhappy too about the lack of community health facilities and programmes in the country as a whole. The Council's recommendations therefore included plans for the introduction of a regional administrative structure for existing hospitals, including systematized referral and co-ordination of hospital and clinic services, and the development of a coherent planning system for hospital facilities and services. At the time more than 70 per cent of all hospitals were in the hands of private owners, and these facilities had developed haphazardly prior to the war; the likelihood of superimposing a rational and systematized approach to their organization stood little chance of success. The opportunity for Japan to start from scratch was therefore, perhaps predictably, lost. Hospital services remained outside the scope and influence of government planning mechanisms and this has had consequences for service provision until the present time. Unable to change very much in the service delivery system the policy-makers turned their attention to the financing of medical care as a means of attaining their goal of equal access to health care for the country. Public health programmes were in the meantime being slowly developed. The Health Centre Law of 1947 charged all prefectural and municipal governments with developing local health bureaux or departments and they were required to set up public health centres providing free services to the public. We shall later see the kinds of provisions which were developed.

The Japanese health care system today remains characterized by the separation in organization and planning of public health programmes and personal medical services; attempts to review or evaluate the appropriateness of this model or to improve co-ordination between the two systems remain sporadic.

During the last few years of the 1940s and during the 1950s, the various health and social insurance schemes, which had started after the National Health Insurance Law of 1938, were expanded to include more and more sectors and occupational groups. By the end of the 1950s with the basic administrative machinery for health and welfare in place, the government could focus more specifically on the inauguration of new social security measures and the improvement of those already in place. With the economy getting back into gear and indeed showing signs of considerable growth Japan was also not unaware of developments taking place in the rest of the world and was still, as ever, anxious to take her place as an equal with the other developed nations of the world. The 1960s and early 1970s can therefore be described with some justification as the golden era of social welfare and social security in Japan. Government policies at this time were an immense improvement on what had gone before; more public funds were made available to improve welfare benefits. In the light of subsequent developments, especially since 1980, it is realistic to assess this period as an aberration from the norm. At heart the concept of the welfare state does not easily accord with either official or popular notions of what is the right course for Japan.

In an attempt to simplify health care financing and make access to medical care easier the New National Health Insurance Law of 1958 was enacted and eventually implemented in 1961. In simple terms this measure introduced universal compulsory health care insurance. However, the insurance carriers remained as diverse and numerous as before and the system today is still quite complicated (in Chapter 5 we describe health care financing in detail). It enjoys widespread popular support and has achieved what it set out to do, as it assures a basic level of health and medical care without imposing undue financial pressure on the individual or family.

There have been critics of course. At one time the labour unions advocated an integrated health insurance scheme covering the whole population; and the single most vociferous critic of the system has been the Japan Medical Association (JMA) which has continued to lobby government, without success, for a single unified scheme. The doctors have never been totally happy with the fee reimbursements, which are an integral part of the health insurance system. In some respects their complaints are justified: the multiplicity of schemes requires prodigious amounts of form-filling and paperwork in the complex billing and reimbursement systems. The activity is labour-intensive, detailed, and complicated; it is only slowly being made easier and more efficient in some of the larger hospitals by the introduction of computerized accounts systems. Individual practitioners and small clinics either continue with outdated manual systems or must bear the costs themselves of any investment in computer hardware which will streamline the process.

Once universal health insurance was in place the government was able to improve coverage, increase the level of benefits by reducing the percentage of co-payment required of dependants, and indeed eventually introduce a ceiling on the total amount of the patient's liability. Government thus subsidized a large share of national medical expenditure out of the central exchequer. Amendments to the National Insurance Law were made in 1966, 1968, and 1973.

Although government policy did not extend to tackling the health service delivery system it did take up the question of medical manpower. It supported the development of a large number of new, mostly private medical schools during the 1960s in order to overcome a shortage of doctors. Positions for the new graduates in the established and larger hospitals were limited but with universal medical insurance fuelling consumer demand for more medical care there was a burgeoning of private clinics and hospitals.

It is ironic that at the beginning of the 1980s Japan had achieved an unlooked-for equality with the advanced industrial nations in the area of health and social welfare expenditure; the major problems facing government bore a remarkable similarity to those of Japan's major political partners and trading competitors. Her policies for health and social welfare are now in a third and possibly most critical phase. The key political issues for Japan in the 1980s have been summarized as the adjustment of foreign and national security policies for an enlarged Japanese role in the international arena, reorganization of the domestic political system and a programme of administrative reform, and financial, economic, and social security policy.[4] Policy for health care, and particularly health care financing, has come under scrutiny as part of these issues.

In order to deal with the issues of social security and finance policy and to evaluate the best ways of implementing changes in administration the government, with the initiative coming from Prime Minister Nakasone, set up the Administrative Reform Council in 1980 under the chairmanship of one of the country's pre-eminent business leaders, Toshiwo Doko, the honorary chairman of Keidanren, the Japan Federation of Economic Organizations. The Council has a number of specialized subcommittees and study groups whose members have been selected from government, business, labour, and academia. The Administrative Reform Council has issued a number of reports, and specific recommendations about health and social welfare have guided the Ministry of Health and Welfare in policy formation as a result. The long-term objectives of administrative reform have as their underlying ideology the creation of 'a dynamic welfare society' which will 'contribute actively to the international community'.[5]

A major LDP preoccupation since the mid-1970s has been to slow down growth in government and to control public spending but it was reluctant to implement what would have been unpopular policies to achieve these ends. When it became clear that the Conservative-led governments in the USA and the UK were embarked on similar programmes of restraint, the government in Japan used overseas examples to its political advantage. Included in the Administrative Reform Council's First Report of 10 July 1981 were recommendations to keep down government expenditure and slash government subsidies by 10 per cent. On medical care the report stated:

> Medical care
> Costs should be borne by the beneficiary where possible. Raise the maximum amount to be paid by beneficiaries of expensive medical treatment. Require elderly beneficiaries to bear part of their medical expenses.

The Third Report of 30 July 1982 again included a specific recommendation related to health care thus

> Social welfare
> Reform public pension schemes to cope with the growing proportion of elderly people. Gradually integrate all public pension schemes. Centralize pension administration. Rationalize medical costs to curb total medical expenditures.

And lastly the Fifth Report of 14 March 1983 notes

> Reform trends
> Transfer one-tenth of government controlled activities to local authorities over the next two years.

And in discussion of the reorganization and rationalization of subsidies which 'need to be strictly curtailed', there is specific reference to the national (i.e. government-sponsored) health insurance system and a need for reinsurance of high medical costs.

Recent government concern and subsequent policy decisions have therefore concentrated on health and medical expenditures and on health care financing mechanisms much to the exclusion of any real attempt to tackle other important factors such as the nature of the health care delivery system, public demand, or the suitability of the kind of health and medical care being provided. What were the main reasons for the relatively new and relatively late – by comparison with the other advanced industrial nations – anxiety about health care expenditure? Compared to other developed countries Japan's national expenditure on medical care as a proportion of total national spending had been low during the 1960s and 1970s when other countries were experiencing hefty increases in the proportion of GNP devoted to health. As we can see from the OECD figures shown in Table 4.1, spending on health care as a proportion of GDP certainly grew in Japan but at nothing like the rate of increase observed in other OECD nations. Moreover average annual growth in national income in Japan during the 1960s was about the same or slightly more than growth in health expenditure. Thus Japan was essentially able to meet the costs of providing health care.

The annual percentage increase in expenditure on health was nevertheless a large one and during the 1960s the percentage

Table 4.1 The share of health expenditure in national expenditure, 1960–83 (percentage of total expenditure on health in GDP)

Country	*1960*	*1965*	*1970*	*1975*	*1980*	*1982*	*1983*
Germany	4.8	5.1	5.6	8.1	8.1	8.2	8.2
Australia	5.1	5.3	5.7	7.6	7.4	7.6	7.5
Austria	4.4	4.7	5.3	6.4	7.0	7.3	7.3
Belgium	3.4	3.9	4.1	5.5	6.3	6.2	6.5
Canada	5.5	6.1	7.2	7.4	7.3	8.2	—
Denmark	3.6	4.8	6.1	6.5	6.8	6.8	6.6
Spain	—	2.7	4.1	5.1	5.9	6.3	—
United States	5.3	6.1	7.6	8.6	9.5	10.6	10.8
Finland	4.2	4.9	5.6	5.8	6.3	6.6	6.6
France	4.3	5.3	6.1	7.6	8.5	9.3	9.3
Greece	2.9	3.1	3.9	4.0	4.2	4.4	4.7
Ireland	4.0	4.4	5.6	7.7	8.7	8.2	—
Iceland	5.9	6.1	8.7	—	7.7	7.6	—
Italy	3.9	4.6	5.5	6.7	6.8	7.2	7.4
Japan	3.0	4.5	4.6	5.7	6.4	6.6	6.7
Luxembourg	—	—	4.9	5.9	6.6	6.5	—
Norway	3.3	3.9	5.0	6.7	6.8	6.8	6.9
New Zealand	4.4	—	4.5	5.2	5.7	5.7	—
Netherlands	3.9	4.4	6.0	7.7	8.3	8.7	8.8
Portugal	—	—	—	6.4	6.1	5.7	—
United Kingdom	3.9	4.2	4.5	5.5	5.8	5.9	6.2
Sweden	4.7	5.6	7.2	8.0	9.5	9.7	9.6
Switzerland	3.3	3.8	5.2	7.1	7.2	7.8	—
Turkey	—	—	—	—	—	—	—
OECD average	4.1	4.7	5.6	6.7	7.2	7.4	7.6

Source: OECD, *Measuring Health Care, 1960–1983: Expenditure, Costs and Performance*, Social Policy Studies 2, Paris, OECD, 1985, p. 12

increase in national medical expenditure each year had been consistently more than 15 per cent. Japan was rather slow to wake up to the implications of the health care cost spiral but did eventually realize that she could not continue to sustain the level of increase she had supported so far – the average annual increase recorded during the 1970s of 18 per cent would lead to a doubling of expenditure every four years. The main reasons for the increase in costs were similar to those experienced in other counties and included

1. rising demand and higher expectations from a more affluent and highly educated population,
2. the introduction of universal health insurance, which fuelled demand as constraints on ability to pay were lifted,
3. a government increase in service fees to the providers, and higher labour costs brought about by pay rises,
4. the beginnings of a massive demographic shift in the population

combined with the provision of free health care for the aged (enacted in 1972, enforced in 1973).

The last factor especially has provided the impetus for major efforts to devise an equitable system of health care financing and service delivery. The impact of a rapidly increasing proportion of elderly people in Japan's population began to be felt in the 1970s. Between 1950 and 1990 Japan will see the proportion of people aged 65 and over jump from 5 per cent to 12 per cent. As of 1983 they comprised 9.7 per cent of the population. It has been projected that by 2025 people aged 65 and over will constitute 21 per cent of the total population as compared to 15.8 per cent in the USA and 18.6 per cent in Britain and France.[7] This critical demographic shift, the so-called greying of society, has been common to all developed countries of course; in Japan however the process got under way rather later and will be effected within a much shorter time-span. Japan will see the number of old people become a substantial proportion of the community far more quickly than has been the case anywhere else in the world to date. The impact of an ageing society in combination with changing patterns of disease dramatically affects health care expenditure and produces an especially onerous burden on public expenditure. In Japan average medical expenses for each person aged 70 or over are approximately triple the per capita medical expenses for the population as a whole. Table 4.2 illustrates the increase in medical expenditure for elderly people in the past ten years. As part of overall policy for the improvement of social welfare provisions in the late 1960s and early 1970s the government had introduced free health care for the aged in 1973; between 1973 and 1974 the largest percentage increase in national medical expenditure – 36.2 per cent – was recorded. The increase in costs was distributed over the many insurance schemes but the largest share fell on the national insurance scheme run by government which has the largest proportion of retirees among its subscribers. Critics of the programme also believed that provision of free treatment encouraged the provision of excessive services by doctors and hospitals and encouraged a lack of awareness about personal responsibility for health care.

Since 1981 therefore the government has attempted to find the right mechanisms to restrain demand for health and medical services without having to resort to the imposition of real limits or cuts in supply. As we have suggested, health policy in its present phase has focused almost exclusively on the health financing system and consideration of the nature of the service delivery system has assumed a secondary role.

Table 4.2 Trends in national medical care costs and medical care costs for the aged

Year	*National medical care costs (100 million yen)*	*Rate of increase (%)*	*Medical care costs for the aged (100 million yen)*	*Rate of increase (%)*	*Ratio of medical care costs for the elderly per national medical care costs*
1974	53,786	36.2	6,652	55.1	12.4
1975	64,779	20.4	8,666	30.3	13.4
1976	76,684	18.4	10,780	24.4	14.1
1977	85,685	11.7	12,872	19.4	15.0
1978	100,042	16.8	15,948	23.9	15.9
1979	109,510	9.5	18,503	16.0	16.9
1980	119,805	9.4	21,269	14.9	17.8
1981	128,709	7.4	24,281	14.2	18.9
1982	138,659	7.9	27,487	13.2	19.8
1983	145,438	4.9	33,185	—	22.8
1984	150,932	3.8	36,098	8.8	23.9

Source: 'Investigation by Department of Health for the Aged', Ministry of Health and Welfare, Outline of Social Insurance in Japan, 1986, Tokyo: Japan International Social Securities Association

> To meet people's increasingly sophisticated and diversified needs for medical care and health promotion services the health insurance system must be up-dated via the well-coordinated combination of medical care covered by insurance benefits and optional care paid for by patients.[8]

This puts in a nutshell the thrust of governmental intentions for future provisions and their payment. Specifically there will be increased levels of co-payment by the insured and their dependants; differential levels of contribution from one scheme to the next will be eradicated. By 1995 each individual will be paying 20 per cent of medical care costs, up to a prescribed ceiling, and insurance medical benefits will be standardized at 80 per cent. (Although not taken into account in the development of government policy a spin-off of this measure is thought to be growth in the market for private health insurance, as families insure themselves to cover the 20 per cent contribution; life assurance companies are starting to prepare suitable packages.) Next, the existing health insurance schemes will be rationalized via mergers of some of the smaller ones. Management of the insurance bodies will be upgraded and operational systems improved through the introduction and use of computer and other technology. In order to exercise some controls on supplier-generated costs tighter monitoring procedures are to be implemented in the fee-reimbursement system; there will be closer scrutiny of doctors' and hospitals' insurance claims to curb over-servicing and over-prescribing and possibly to monitor quality of service. The point-fee system itself is to be streamlined and simplified; this is likely to be welcomed by many service-providers in the interests of reducing the administrative and clerical costs associated with the filing of claims. Use of new, highly costly technology will be reimbursed only in approved facilities, thus cutting down the indiscriminate spread of such equipment throughout all levels of service-providers.

Drug prices have already received a lot of official attention and are now more strictly controlled than in the 1960s and 1970s; the list price for many products has been cut and there will be much tighter systems for monitoring drug prescriptions. However the existing system of independent negotiation and purchase by individual clinics and hospitals leaves pricing by the manufacturers open to some manipulation.

In so far as the government has devoted any attention to the nature and quality of health care offered, policy measures confirm that the status quo will not be fundamentally changed. The government appears to be fully aware of the deficiencies in the present system, of the problems inherent in a system which is not a system at all but a loose and uncontrolled set of facilities and services, which are not co-ordinated and for which there is no centralized body with responsibility for planning and management. The government has declared that 'well-defined function and role sharing must be realized among various medical care facilities from clinics to advanced specialised hospitals' and that 'priority must be placed on primary care'.[9] However, quite how its stated goals are to be achieved is not yet evident in any concrete fashion in plans formulated to date.

Amendments to the Medical Service Law in 1983 proposed regional medical care planning and required the prefectures to develop co-ordinated medical care plans and strategies. As of 1989 all of the forty-seven prefectures had managed to produce a plan; the focus of regional planning remains hospitals and bed numbers. Reference is made to the construction of a functional and operational network among hospitals and clinics, but given the independence of these facilities the establishment of a formally co-ordinated service is difficult to envisage.

The government is concerned, as we have seen, about primary care and is keen to see some changes in the nature of medical practice; it sees private medical practitioners becoming family physicians rather than providing diluted or poor-quality specialist services. Government initiatives in this area have had a lukewarm response from the medical practitioners, many considering that such a move will devaluc their services in the public eye and constitute a threat to their income; the Japan Medical Association's endorsement which could swing things the government's way is not yet forthcoming. Among the medical profession at large the prevailing attitude remains that medical services exist to tackle and cure sickness and that provision of preventive services is for somebody else to take care of. The government has secured the profession's agreement regarding the future supply of doctors and it has been agreed that the number of entrants to medical schools will be reduced by 10 per cent per annum until 1995 in order to avoid creating a surplus of doctors.

Some facilities at present operated by the national government are to be off-loaded on to prefectural and local governments – another method of reducing the national government's share of total health expenditure.

To recap then, the core of Japan's health policy for the coming ten to fifteen years is to maintain access and to ensure the provision of acceptable and adequate health care with a well-defined sharing of the total costs between the government, the insurers, and the consumers. All the evidence suggests that the public is satisfied with cost-sharing and is not averse to making some payment at point of service; in a society which has traditionally stressed the need for personal responsibility the government's approach to payment of services is not a contentious issue. Whether, or indeed if, this approach can properly provide the most suitable kinds of services for elderly or chronically sick people is still a matter of debate and concern.

The policy-making process

So far in this chapter we have presented an outline of the political and historical context of health policy in Japan up until the present. We have seen how the focus of official health policy has evolved in the past one hundred years and we have learned too that contemporary health policy issues in Japan are strikingly similar to those in other advanced industrial nations. The ways in which Japan is tackling these issues are, not surprisingly, dissimilar in a number of key ways from the kinds of solutions or approaches being considered elsewhere. This is perhaps as it should be.

In identifying the main features of current health policy we have touched on the work of the Administrative Reform Council and its critical role in all aspects of the government's (essentially however the Liberal Democratic Party) goal of achieving national administrative reform. What we now need to explore is the policy process in Japan: how are national-level decisions reached and subsequently translated into local-level action? We will consider first the Ministry of Health and Welfare, its organization, functions, and its role in the health policy process; the nature and role of the key political instruments, the Diet, ministers, civil servants, and representatives of interested pressure groups and community representatives.

Koseisho, the Ministry of Health and Welfare

The Ministry of Health and Welfare, Koseisho, was established in 1938 and reconstituted in 1949; the ministry is responsible at the national level for the general administration of public health, social welfare, and social security programmes. Organizationally it consists of the minister's Secretariat, nine bureaux, the Social Insurance Agency, and a number of affiliated specialist research institutes or national service institutions. The present organization chart of the ministry is shown in Figure 4.1. Most directly concerned with health and medical care provisions are a number of bodies. The *Minister's Secretariat*, which is in charge of overall planning, fundamental policy co-ordination of programmes, and liaison with the Diet, Cabinet, and Prime Minister's office. It conducts public information programmes on health and welfare administration.

The *Health Policy Bureau*, newly established in 1984 as a result of recommendations from one of the specialist Administrative Reform Council subcommittees, has overall responsibility for the planning and promotion of comprehensive policy in the field of prevention, health care, and rehabilitation, and achieves a separation of health policy-making from the supervisory functions of the various bureaux. The *Health Service Bureau* manages the national hospitals and sanatoria and is in charge of monitoring and surveillance of communicable and infectious diseases. The *Department of Health for the Aged* is also a new unit set up within this Bureau in 1982 and is responsible, as the name suggests, for policy, planning, and supervision of health and medical care programmes for elderly people.

The *Environmental Health Bureau* has jurisdiction over sanitation, hygiene, and sanitation standards in public facilities and through the *Water Supply and Environmental Sanitation Department* authority over the maintenance of clean water supplies and the proper disposal of waste. A separate government body, the Environmental Agency set up in 1971, is not a part of Koseisho and is concerned with environmental pollution and protection, monitoring, surveillance, and enforcement of some of the strictest anti-pollution measures and regulations in the world. The *Pharmaceutical Affairs Bureau* enforces a massively complex system of regulations for the manufacture, import, and sales of drugs, cosmetics, and medical devices to ensure safety and efficacy.

The *Health Insurance Bureau* is in charge of planning and operation of National Health Insurance, monitoring of medical fees, and establishment of scales for service charges. It also supervises the activities of the health insurance societies. The *Medical and Child Health Division of the Children and Families Bureau* is responsible for making policies on maternal and child health programmes, including family planning, providing financial aid, and supervising programmes in the prefectures and municipalities.

The *Statistics and Information Department*, in addition to compiling and analysing routine health and vital statistics, carries out a series of regular annual national health related surveys. These obtain data on medical and health services demand, health insurance, and medical care costs and benefits; updates on medical care facilities, health centre activity reports; health manpower statistics, such as the number of physicians, dentists, nurses, and allied health personnel and their distribution and type of employment. It also collects school health, maternal and child health, and industrial health statistics.

Each bureau has its own planning and research functions and also provides grants to academic and other institutions for research and development. Formerly too the bureaux developed their own policy specifically for their special area; with the establishment of the Health Policy Bureau a more centralized and co-ordinated approach to health policy formulation has been undertaken. Not under the aegis of the Ministry of Health and Welfare is the school health programme, which is the responsibility of the Ministry of Education, which has decentralized authority for school health programmes to the prefectures and local authorities. Likewise industrial health programmes are administered by the Labour Health section of the Labour Standard Bureau of the Ministry of Labour. This function has not however been decentralized.

Apart from the management of national hospitals and sanatoria and of the specialist centres such as the National Heart Centre and the National Cardiovascular Disease Centre, the ministry is not involved in the provision of health care services. Public health care provisions are in the hands of prefectural and local government authorities.

Local governments

The present system of public administration in Japan goes back to the modernization programme carried out during the Meiji Restoration and also contains some characteristics from the system of local

Figure 4.1 Organization chart of the Ministry of Health and Welfare, 1988

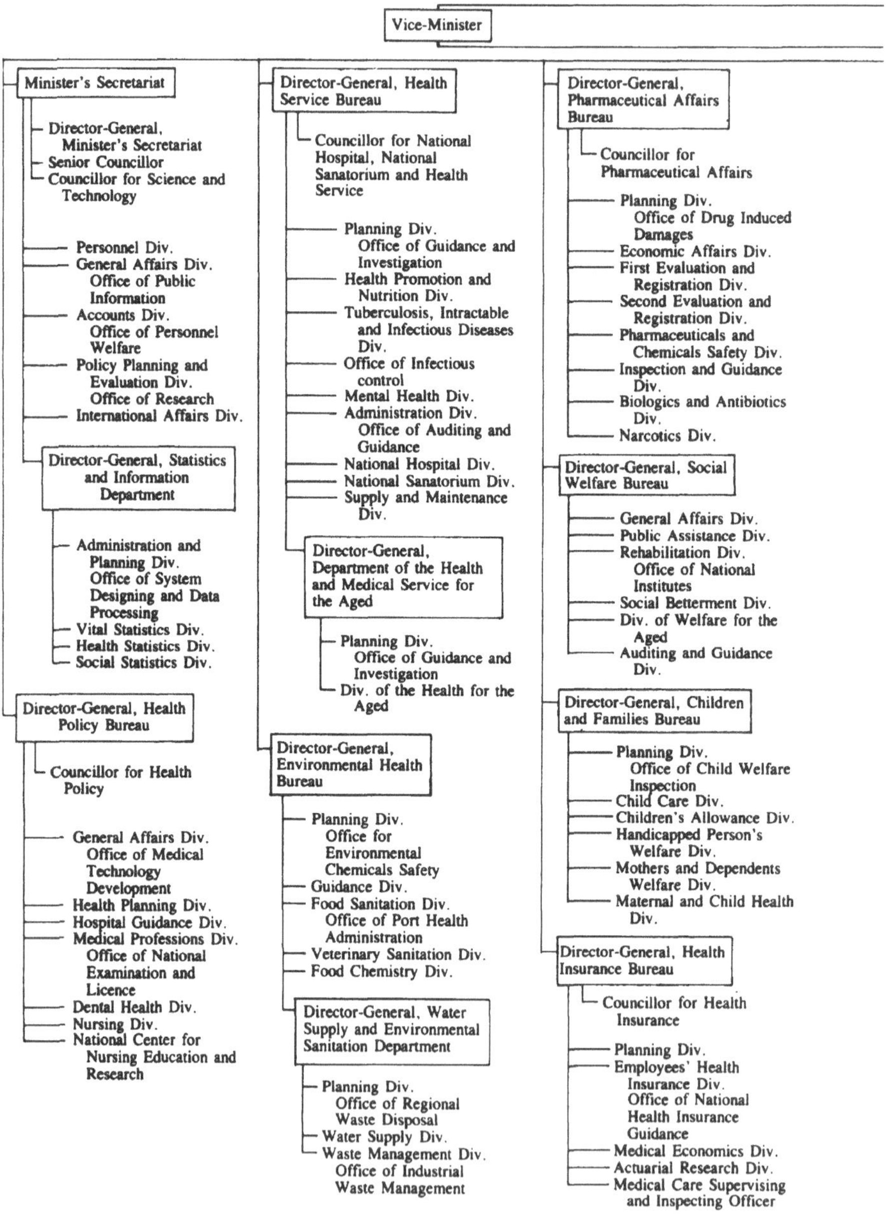

Source: Health and Welfare Services in Japan, 1988. Ministry of Health and Welfare, Tokyo: Japan International Corporation of Welfare Services.

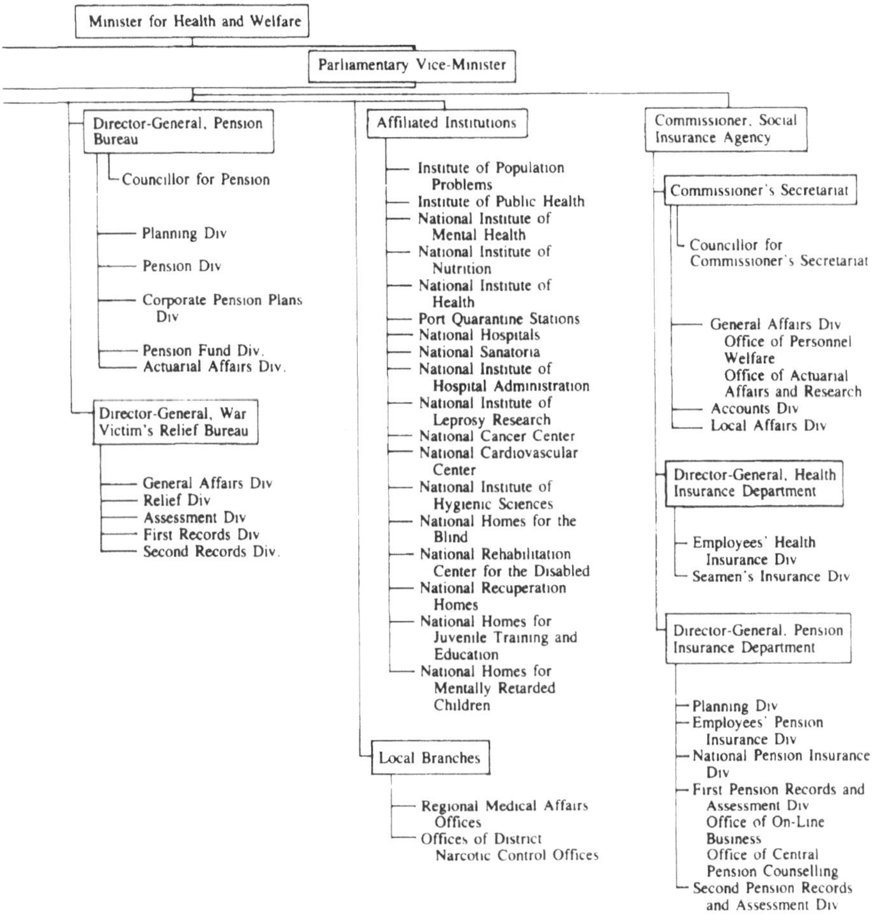
Minister for Health and Welfare
Parliamentary Vice-Minister
Director-General, Pension Bureau
Councillor for Pension
Planning Div
Pension Div
Corporate Pension Plans Div
Pension Fund Div.
Actuarial Affairs Div.
Director-General, War Victim's Relief Bureau
General Affairs Div
Relief Div
Assessment Div
First Records Div
Second Records Div.
Affiliated Institutions
Institute of Population Problems
Institute of Public Health
National Institute of Mental Health
National Institute of Nutrition
National Institute of Health
Port Quarantine Stations
National Hospitals
National Sanatoria
National Institute of Hospital Administration
National Institute of Leprosy Research
National Cancer Center
National Cardiovascular Center
National Institute of Hygienic Sciences
National Homes for the Blind
National Rehabilitation Center for the Disabled
National Recuperation Homes
National Homes for Juvenile Training and Education
National Homes for Mentally Retarded Children
Local Branches
Regional Medical Affairs Offices
Offices of District Narcotic Control Offices
Commissioner, Social Insurance Agency
Commissioner's Secretariat
Councillor for Commissioner's Secretariat
General Affairs Div
Office of Personnel Welfare
Office of Actuarial Affairs and Research
Accounts Div
Local Affairs Div
Director-General, Health Insurance Department
Employees' Health Insurance Div
Seamen's Insurance Div
Director-General, Pension Insurance Department
Planning Div
Employees' Pension Insurance Div
National Pension Insurance Div
First Pension Records and Assessment Div
Office of On-Line Business
Office of Central Pension Counselling
Second Pension Records and Assessment Div

government of the feudal times. The main unit in regional organization of the country is the prefecture, of which there are forty-seven, each with its own capital city, elected assembly, and government offices. As far as health care administration is concerned each prefectural government has a department or bureau which is responsible for planning and carrying out health programmes in compliance with the policies and directions of the ministry.

After the prefectures come the primary local authorities – the city, town and village governments (see Figure 4.2 for an illustration of the system). These authorities similarly have a division or section in charge of health, and are responsible for planning and implementing public health care programmes at the appropriate local government levels. Under the Health Centre Law of 1947 for example, prefectures are required to establish public health centres; the National Insurance Law of 1961 required local governments to establish and run health insurance programmes, and many local insurance bodies in fact own and operate, or manage medical care facilities. For a number of years too the central body, the Ministry of Health and Welfare, has endorsed the concept of integrated health planning by local authorities. There are problems with implementation however, as local authorities have no real jurisdiction over the bulk of the medical service-providers in their area of authority who are the private practitioners, hospitals, and clinics. The nature and level of local authority provisions consequently vary greatly from one authority to the next; the commonest pattern of planning appears to be the establishment of 'advisory' committees, with membership drawn from the local branch of the JMA, voluntary organizations, education authorities, social welfare agencies, and of course the local government health centre or health department employees.[10]

The bureaucracy

The political head of Koseisho is the Minister for Health and Welfare, a Diet and Cabinet member and for the past thirty-five years this position has been held by an LDP member. Up until 1986 the then Minister of Health and Welfare was a strong supporter of the present Prime Minister and a staunch advocate of policies to curb government expenditure on health care; it is undoubtedly through his efforts that the recommendations of the Administrative Reform Council have taken on the nature they have. The leading roles in the drama of policy-making in Japan are taken by the bureaucrats, to an extent that their counterparts elsewhere would envy. As Yanaga notes:

Figure 4.2 Japan: system of public administration

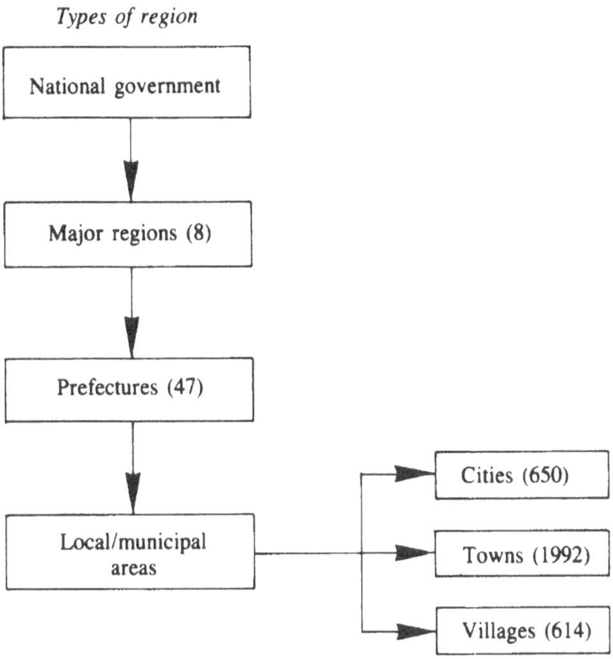

Source: D. MacDonald, *A Geography of Modern Japan*, Paul Norbury Publications Ltd, 1985, p. 148

> Their political masters, including the cabinet ministers, decide only the broadest outlines of policy, leaving the implementation entirely to the permanent administrators. The higher civil servants are therefore the 'permanent politicians'. They effectively control the administrative machinery and are intensely jealous of their autonomy. Politicians often lay down policy regarding the status, composition and operations of an administrative agency, but its execution is always left to the civil servants, who always have the last say and who invariably get their way.[11]

Things change but slowly, if at all, in Japan. The by-now apparently permanent establishment of the same political masters, working with civil servants who are also employed for life, ensures that policy development, or evolution, proceeds smoothly without the kind of hiccups which occur when a new government enters office. As a result policies are generally acceptable to all interested parties; equally they tend to be bland and achieve change only incrementally. Many policies are merely guidelines or vague recommendations and interpretations and implementation are very much up to the bureaucracy, which invariably does what it wants to do.

Japan has a long history of executive supremacy and provisions of the post-war Constitution notwithstanding, the bureaucracy still has massive, all-pervasive power. It is the case that in many countries the civil service offers, to all but a high-flying few, scant financial reward compared to business or industry, very little status, and even less public respect. In Japan on the contrary the civil service continues to attract and indeed is actively sought by the best graduates of the country's leading universities. The attractions of the civil services are not especially the material rewards – although financial security and steady progress are in fact assured – but prestige, respect, and power. The graduate entrant will move upwards through the ranks, gradually acquiring seniority and amassing more power as he does so, and influence which extends beyond the ministry walls.

The bureaucrats consider themselves the watchdogs of the national interest and are esteemed as such by the general public. They are central to policy-making and a decisive influence in how it is implemented. Without a real parliamentary opposition the Diet is often little more than a polite debating chamber and it has little or no power to veto bureaucracy-inspired legislation. Cabinet members act to channel departmental proposals from the ministry to the Diet. The bureaucracy is in the key position for producing the legislative programme which the Cabinet submits to the Diet and the ministries prepare the Bills. Even if an individual Diet member manages to get a Bill into the Diet for debate, the Bill more often than not is the result of the work of bureaucrats, depending on the scope of the Diet members' contacts within the relevant ministry. Many senior civil servants spend considerable amounts of time in the Diet answering members' questions on behalf of the proposing minister or member.

Politicians and civil servants maintain good and close working relationships. Many politicians have come from the ranks of the bureaucracy and therefore understand how it works and appreciate its capabilities; they hold it in some respect and appreciate the value of having the bureaucrats working with them rather than against them.

There are similarly warm relationships between bureaucrats and leaders of commerce, industry, banking, and other private or public bodies; such relationships are actively cultivated in order to ensure continued smooth progression of policy-making and implementation. All the individuals tend to come from the same educational and social background and a mutuality of interests is not difficult to establish and maintain. The influence of a senior official often extends long after his official term of office expires because of the tradition of appointing 'retired' civil servants to 'honorary' but powerful positions in quasi-governmental agencies or affiliated institutions. In what is known as the 'descent from heaven' senior civil servants may leave a ministry to take up high-ranking positions in private industry after they have attained the highest possible position within their ministry and further promotion is not possible as the number of positions available is fewer than the number of suitable senior-level staff.

The supremacy of the bureaucracy in policy-making does not mean that other groups do not contribute to or influence official policy. Take the case of health policy: by and large the research institutions affiliated with the Ministry of Health and Welfare enjoy academic freedom and individual staff members in such organizations may be widely known for their dissenting views. However as the heads of such organizations are often former civil servants the views of the ministry will be clearly communicated to the institute's staff and subsequent reports and recommendations will tend to echo ministry requirements. The research institutes provide the necessary statistical back-up and background documentation for policy and planning issues and at the end of the day will produce findings of sufficient neutrality not to raise any bureaucratic eyebrows. The government and its various departments make considerable use too of officially appointed committees and study groups, who are usually given precise briefs in order to guide them in their work and in their final conclusions.

Bureaucrats also view politicians with a fair degree of respect; bureaucrats may well be conscious of their supremacy but they are not unappreciative of the public influence of politicians and of their value in communications. They frequently consult with Diet members to obtain a sounding for policy proposals; civil servants certainly make it their business to know which parliamentarians are most influential within any of the party factions, which ones are on the up and up, and which ones are fading powers. Each political party and the parliamentary committees have full-time specialists who serve as *de facto* advisers to the Diet members. Among parliamentary privileges is the right of investigation by which Diet members can require ministry staff to provide data and information on any issue.

Government provisions for health care

In Japan as elsewhere social, economic, and demographic changes have led to greater government concern and involvement in a number of areas of health care. There is in Japan however considerable functional, institutional, and territorial fragmentation of responsibility for health care provision so that the application of coherent policies and planning instruments to affect overall provisions is difficult. Government policy is to continue to rely on the private sector for the provision of hospital and primary medical services in order to keep a lid on public sector costs. At the same time there is some recognition of a need for input by government agencies in critical areas which cannot be well served by the private sector. Government has taken an overall responsibility for a few areas (e.g. pharmaceutical affairs), directs the programmes, or provides limited subsidies to local governments to implement suitable programmes. Through affiliated institutes the national government finances research, provides facilities for selected medical problems, and encourages the development of centres of excellence.

Prefectural and municipal governments are required by law to establish public health centres and these are administered by the local health department or bureau and financed by a mixture of national and local government funds. As of 1985 there were 855 health centres in operation throughout the country: 650 established by prefectural governments and located either in prefectural capitals or other urban centres within the prefecture; 157 health centres are sponsored by municipalities and 53 by the Ward Offices (the equivalent of the London Boroughs) of Metropolitan Tokyo.[12] The intention of the original plan was that there should be one health centre for 100,000 population; development of facilities has not been uniform however, and the larger centres have a catchment population of 250,000 to 300,000. Health centres provide community health services and function as the district health administration unit. Staff therefore include physicians who usually work part-time on a clinic session basis and are responsible for clinical work and the co-ordination of the activities of nursing and allied health staff; public health nurses and midwives, laboratory and X-ray technicians, nutritionists, statisticians, health educators, food, sanitary and meat inspectors. The exact make-up of each centre's personnel varies according to its size and programme. Public health centres have a wide-ranging brief of responsibilities and develop appropriate services for the local population. Programmes range over control of communicable diseases; control and prevention of TB, venereal and other diseases; maternal and child health; consultation on family planning, contraception and abortion; dental care and hygiene; rabies prevention; maintenance of environmental sanitation, provision of public health and home nursing services, advice and guidance on benefits; health laboratory services; and health education programmes. The smaller centres offer a much more limited programme of services and facilities.

The operation and management of community health programmes is the responsibility of prefectural and local governments which have considerable autonomy; the Ministry of Health and Welfare has few statutory instruments to enforce the implementation of recommended guidelines; guidelines are precisely that and national government subsidies must usually be matched by local government contributions so local governments always carry a proportion of programme costs. Naturally the programmes and the commitment to public health provisions vary from one locality to the next. Moreover the nature of the health system is such that interested parties and pressure groups at local level may be influential enough to exert considerable sway over local developments. In rural areas in particular there are shortages of physicians willing to work in public health centres; nurse staffing also remains a difficulty. National government plans therefore to expand the health centre network to 4,000 centres by 1988 are unlikely to be successful.

The development of public maternal and child health (MCH) services is instructive for the light it throws on the policy-making process and the workings of the mechanisms to implement national policy at local levels. The changes which have taken place in this public programme provide a fine example of the role and influence of politically strong pressure groups on health care policy.

By comparison with most other advanced industrialized nations Japan was late in appreciating the importance of proper health care for pregnant women, mothers, and young children. Provisions prior to 1945 were minimal and it was only in the 1950s, when the infant mortality-rate and the maternal mortality-rate were among the highest in the world, that the government was finally forced to do something to improve the situation. (Infant mortality-rates 1950: Japan 60.1 per 1,000, Sweden 21 per 1,000, USA 29.2 per 1,000; maternal mortality-rates 1950: Japan 176 per 100,000 births, USA 83.3 per 100,000 births, Sweden 61.5 per 100,000 births.)

In 1958 the then Permanent Vice-Minister for Health and Welfare issued guidelines for the establishment of MCH centres to the prefectural governments; municipal mayors were advised to request government subsidies to construct MCH centres. Each municipality was to be responsible for the construction of its MCH centre, with the national and prefectural governments each contributing one-third of construction costs, leaving the municipality to cover the remaining one-third. Government policy envisioned a network of MCH centres in rural areas where, in the shortage or absence of medical practitioners, the need to improve maternal and child health was paramount. The construction of purpose-built centres got under way in 1958 and continued steadily throughout the 1960s. There were 405 centres by 1965 when the Maternal and Child Health Law was passed; from the late 1960s onwards however the number of newly constructed or purpose-built centres has been dropping for reasons which we shall describe shortly.

In the early days the MCH programme emphasized the provision of midwifery services. In the 1950s more than 90 per cent of all births in Japan took place at home. Rural women in particular gave birth in poor conditions and they rarely had any antenatal care. Most rural families were not covered by health insurance and thus had to bear the full cost of any medical treatment, which few could afford to do. Diet and nutrition were also poor; in a farming family women were expected to be back at their household and farm chores within a couple of days of giving birth. MCH centres located closer to rural communities meant that women could more easily receive regular antenatal check-ups; more importantly the MCH centres provided facilities for a safe birth, usually attended by a skilled midwife or a doctor in the case of a difficult delivery. Women could stay in the MCH centre for a week or so after delivery, thus obtaining the necessary rest and obtaining help and advice for the care of their babies and themselves in the postpartum period. Delivery and postpartum care were not free but the charges were approximately one-third those of the hospital or private maternity clinic in the nearby town. It has been estimated that 20–30 per cent of women delivering in MCH clinics received financial assistance.[13] In addition to antenatal care and delivery services the centres also provided infant check-ups, including vaccinations, counselling on family planning, and classes in health, hygiene, and child care. These services were free of charge.

Welcomed though the MCH centres were by the users, their existence and the services they have provided have never been entirely accepted by the medical profession. One result has been almost permanent problems in staffing the centres. The centres were set up without any clearly defined criteria for admission of women for delivery and procedures for handling complicated causes were not well spelled out. MCH centres were government-run units: with no real co-ordination between services run by the local authority and the private sector medical facilities, occasional problems arose in the handling of complicated cases. This was a continuing source of tension which finally prompted the ministry to set up a study group in 1966. Membership consisted of representatives of the Japan Medical Association, the Japan Association for Maternal and Child Welfare (a national organization of obstetricians and gynaecologists, and the only group licensed to perform abortions), the Japan Child Health Association, the Japan Midwives Association, the National

Association of Municipalities, and the All-Japan Federation of MCH Centres. The outcome of the study was an amendment to the rules governing the nature of MCH centres and the location within the municipality or district. Priority was shifted from midwifery services to the provision of health guidance. It was determined that plans for the development of new MCH centres required prior consultation between the local government and the local branch of the JMA. Originally local governments had been at liberty to set up MCH centres where they assessed the need as being greatest. In 1974 a further amendment by the Ministry of Health and Welfare allowed for the provision of national government subsidies for centres providing general MCH and health programmes without the midwifery component.

As the authors of the 'History of MCH' centres point out, 'both of the above-mentioned points aimed to establish a harmonious relationship with medical associations. As a consequence of the amendment the number of newly established MCH centres has declined since 1968'.[14] The medical profession's reservations and dissatisfaction with the MCH centres focused primarily on their role in delivery (in 1965 12 per cent of all deliveries took place in MCH centres and clinics) and it is significant that these reservations came to the fore at a time when MCH centres were providing a fairly large sector of the population with a service which the private medical practitioners and hospitals were not. There is no doubt that clinical considerations played a part in the medical association's stand but it is equally certain that the impact of the MCH centre's free services on the income of the medical practitioners was also an issue. In the mid-1960s the JMA was engaged in continuous and often bitter dispute with the government over fee schedules and the ruling on MCH centres was a valuable bargaining point for the government to gain JMA concessions on fees and for continued JMA support of other policies and programmes.

Health services for elderly people

The provision of acceptable and appropriate health care services for the rapidly growing number of elderly people in the population is now a critical element in government policy. Official concern grew because of the dramatic rise both in the absolute cost of medical care for elderly people and in the ratio of medical care costs for the elderly to total national medical care costs. Thus in 1973 medical care costs for the aged were 4,289 million yen (10.8 per cent of national medical care costs) and jumped by 55 per cent in the following year after the introduction of free services; by 1983 total medical

Table 4.3 Trends in the ratio of medical care costs for the aged (%)

Year	*Government-managed health insurance*	*Society-managed health insurance*	*Mutual aid associations*	*Day labourers' health insurance*	*Seamen's insurance*	*National health insurance*	*All medical care insurance*
1974	7.7	8.6	12.4	6.2	11.0	23.0	14.3
1975	8.8	9.6	13.6	6.7	12.1	24.2	15.5
1976	9.3	10.1	14.5	7.0	12.6	25.0	16.2
1977	10.0	10.8	15.3	7.4	13.5	26.3	17.2
1978	10.6	11.4	15.6	8.0	14.6	27.7	18.3
1979	11.1	11.8	16.1	8.5	15.9	29.1	19.2
1980	11.6	11.9	15.9	9.1	16.4	30.5	20.0
1981	12.4	12.5	16.8	9.5	17.7	32.0	21.2
1982	13.2	12.9	17.2	16.1	12.4	33.1	22.2
1983	16.8	14.6	17.6	21.6	20.0	37.4	25.7

Source: 'Investigation by Department of Health for the Aged', Ministry of Health and Welfare, *Outline of Social Insurance in Japan*, 1986, Tokyo: Japan International Social Services Association

Note: These ratios are calculated based on medical care costs from April of one year to March of the next.

care costs for elderly people were 33,185 million yen and accounted for 22.8 per cent of national medical spending (see Table 4.2).

Alarm about these figures was all the greater because government-managed health insurance schemes insured a disproportionate number of elderly people. In 1980 for example only 9 per cent of National Health Insurance members were elderly but their medical expenses accounted for more than 30 per cent of NHI expenses. The society-managed insurance schemes had fewer elderly members and were paying out just over 12 per cent in benefits for this age group. Government was obviously most affected by the rise in health care costs for this sector of the population (see Table 4.3).

We saw earlier that the provision of free medical care for elderly people introduced in 1973 had not been wholeheartedly welcomed by many of those involved in health care, hence the revisions under the Health and Medical Services for the Elderly Act of August 1982 (and enforced February 1983) were well received. To date there has been no consumer research or any official attempt to establish the impact of the revised provisions on the recipients and users: elderly people themselves.

The Act introduced co-payment by elderly people for medical care and has as its goal the realization of a co-ordinated health activities programme involving sickness prevention, treatment, and rehabilitation. In keeping with government policy, actual provisions are left

Figure 4.3 International comparison of preferred relationship with children and grandchildren

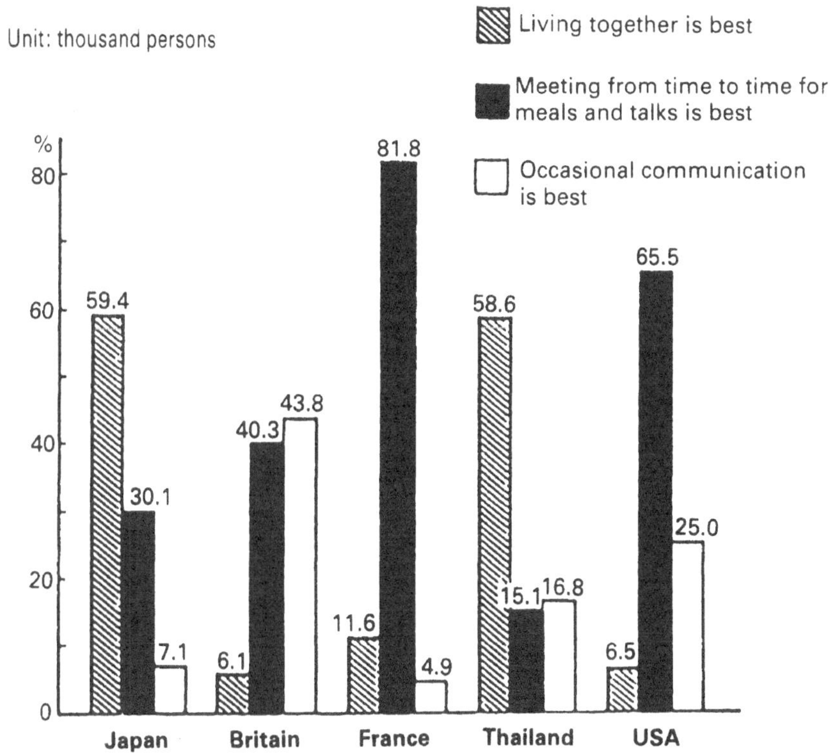

Source: Japan's Rapidly Aging Population, Foreign Press Centre, Reference Reading Series, No. 9, Tokyo, 1982

to the discretion of the prefectural or local authority health department. The system is financed by national, prefectural, and local authority contributions and individuals must of course pay premiums. Medical benefits include physician consultations, supply of medicines and other therapeutic materials, hospitalization, surgery, and other necessary therapy or treatment, nursing, and transportation. The individual's co-payment is 500 yen per month for out-patient treatment and 1,000 yen per day for in-patient treatment. On the preventive health side, local authorities are to implement a health promotion and health education programme, which includes an annual health screening and check-up, distribution of a personal health notebook, and health education programmes.

Implementation of the new co-ordinated health services has been patchy and none of the measures is designed to tackle effectively such problems as the long-term care of the chronic elderly sick, bedridden patients, and those in need of full-time nursing care. Some local authorities have started home-nursing programmes but they are not widely available and patients are required to pay a monthly charge; as the primary medical care services remain the responsibility of private practitioners, co-ordination and follow-up also remain difficult. In 1983 there were just over 4,000 facilities for the aged, 63 per cent of which were residential and offered 190,952 places.[15] A further 1,500 welfare centres provided day care, rehabilitation, physiotherapy, and other services. Given that the total population aged 65 and over in 1983 was 11,672 million and those aged 70 and over numbered 7,601 million, it is clear that the number of places is inadequate and the shortfall would be more devastating were it not for the fact that the majority of elderly sick people are still cared for in their own homes by their family, who continue to regard it as their duty. In 1983 more than 65 per cent of people aged 65 and over lived with their children; some 21.3 per cent of elderly married couples lived independently and 9.1 per cent were living alone. The high percentage of parents living with their children is characteristic of Japan; the normal practice is that they live with the eldest son and his wife. Although the numbers of old people living alone is growing each year, the overwhelming preference is still to live with the children (see Figure 4.3). It is largely thanks to the continuation of traditional practices that the poor development of community care and nursing services has not been so ruinous as it might have been. When care of the chronic sick or bedridden patients is necessary the family has only its own resources and financial reserves to fall back on: it is usually the daughter or daughter-in-law who must shoulder the greatest burden of care.

References

1 O. Reischauer, *Japan: The Story of a Nation*, Tokyo, C.E. Tuttle, 1976, p. 140.
2 W.G. Beasley (ed.), *Modern Japan: Aspects of History, Literature and Society*, Tokyo, C.E. Tuttle, 1976; London, Allen and Unwin, 1975, p. 15.
3 J. Ohmura, 'Overview of Japanese Health Insurance', *Japan=Hospitals* 2, p. 17, July 1983.
4 K. Uchida, 'Japanese politics in the 1980s', in R. Shiratori (ed.) *Japan in the 1980s*, Tokyo, New York, and San Francisco, Kodansha International, 1982, p. 63.
5 *Administrative Reform in Japan*, Tokyo, Foreign Press Centre Japan,

1984, pp. 8–9.

6 Ibid, pp. 14, 21, 32–3.

7 N. Yashiro, 'Perspectives on the Aging Society', in *Japan's Rapidly Aging Population*, Tokyo, Foreign Press Centre Japan, 1982, p. 6.

8 *Outline of Recent Japanese Policy on Health: The Background and Measures for Reform*, Ministry of Health and Welfare Paper for Joint Japanese–OECD Conference on Health and Pensions Policies in the Context of Demographic Evolution and Economic Restraint, Tokyo, November 1985, p. 19.

9 *Outline of Recent Japanese Policy on Health*, p. 22.

10 M. Hashimoto, 'Health services in Japan', in M.W. Raffel (ed.) *Comparative Health Systems: Descriptive Analyses of Fourteen National Health Systems*, Philadelphia, Penn, and London, Pennsylvania State University Press, 1984, p. 357.

11 C. Yanaga, *Big Business in Japanese Politics*, New Haven, Conn., in J. Livingstone, J. Moore, and F. Oldfeather (eds) *The Japan Reader: Vol. II Postwar Japan: 1945 to the Present*, New York, Random House and Harmondsworth, Penguin, 1973, p. 420.

12 *Health and Welfare Services in Japan, 1986*, Ministry of Health and Welfare, Tokyo, March 1986, p. 17.

13 *A Twenty Year History of Maternal and Child Health Centers*, Document Series 7, *Japanese Organization for International Co-operation in Family Planning, Inc.* Tokyo, 1982, p. 25. This publication is a valuable source of much information and statistical data referred to in this section.

14 Ibid.

15 *Health and Welfare Statistics in Japan, 1985*, Health and Welfare Statistics Association, Tokyo, 1985, p. 117.

Chapter five

Financing health care

In this chapter we consider both sides of the coin of health care finances in Japan today: spending on health and medical care – the total amount, its growth over the years, and major items of expenditure – and the sources of health care funds. The way in which a country organizes and finances her health care system reflects the values and ideals of that society and its political recognition, transmitted in policy, about what health care is supposed to achieve for its people. In looking at the financial arrangements for health and medical care in Japan we aim to present a clear and detailed picture of the mechanisms employed by government to ensure that policies are successfully implemented and acceptable to the public, and medical care providers.

Health Services expenditure is one of the largest and fastest growing items of social expenditure in the developed countries today. Governments of all political shades and opinion in countries which have developed different and varied health care systems have, in the past decade especially, been attempting to achieve greater control of health care spending. The mechanisms that have been devised and employed to this end have been as varied as the health care systems themselves and in some countries the process has resulted in a major shift in ideology, or fundamental change in the health system. In its detailed study of health expenditure among member countries the OECD notes that much of the growth in health care spending took place in the 1960s, when the economic climate was favourable to expansion in public spending.[1] More stringent economic realities in the 1970s and 1980s have led to the design and implementation of policies which have as their principal goal the control of costs; at the same time financial policies have had to be designed to ensure that access to health care is not denied to citizens. For, as the OECD reports, 'Without mastery of the cost problem, the economic and social trade-offs will be onerous and unacceptable.'[2]

Japan was relatively slow and some way behind other developed countries in introducing cost-containment policies as the government was caught unawares by massive increases in health care costs in the 1970s. Since the beginning of the 1980s cost containment plus equity in access to acceptable standards of medical care have formed the lynchpin of government health care policy. Let us look therefore at how Japan is trying to achieve mastery of the cost problem now and for the future. Japanese efforts to tackle the issue may be instructive.

Japan's social security system encompasses health, pension, and employment security, workmen's accident compensation, and social welfare programmes which provide means-tested cash benefits for elderly and disabled people and other disadvantaged groups. The greatest efforts to streamline and simplify the system took place after the Second World War, but the whole social security system has continued to evolve on a piecemeal basis and this is evident still in the complexity and multiplicity of schemes which are a part of it. Public assistance has remained in essence a back-up for inadequacies in the various health, pension, and employment insurance programmes and is not aimed at equity in income redistribution. Despite considerable growth in absolute and relative terms the scale of social security in Japan for instance remains low by comparison with other developed countries and Japan has the lowest incidence of taxation and social security contribution, as is illustrated in Table 5.1.

Table 5.1 International comparison of tax and social security incidence (%)

	Incidence of taxation	*Incidence of social security payments*	*Total*
Japan (1980)	23.4	9.3	32.7
Britain (1979)	39.3	9.7	49.0
France (1979)	29.3	25.3	54.6
Sweden (1979)	45.1	19.0	64.1
USA (1978)	28.9	9.6	38.5
W. Germany (1979)	32.6	19.6	52.2

Sources: Kokumin Keizai Keisan Nenpo, 'Annual Report on National Economy Accounts', Economic Planning Agency, 1982; *National Accounts of OECD Countries*, Organization for Economic Co-operation and Development
Note: Ratios to national income.

The low ratio is the result of two factors: a small proportion of elderly people in the population and the relatively recent creation of pension plans, most of which started only in 1961.[3]

Rapid economic growth in the 1960s encouraged the improvement of existing social security provisions and the inauguration of new ones. Unfortunately official commitment to upgrade welfare provisions – 1973 saw the introduction of more generous welfare and pension

Table 5.2 Trends in social security benefits, 1970, 1975, 1980, 1982

Fiscal year	*Social security benefits (billion yen)*							
	Medical care	*% of total*	*Pension*	*% of total*	*Others*	*% of total*	*Total*	*National income*
1970	2,075.8	58.9	856.2	24.3	592.0	16.8	3,523.9	60,875.4
1975	5,688.1	48.7	3,931.6	33.7	2,052.9	17.6	11,672.6	123,184.3
1980	10,658.2	43.3	10,470.9	42.6	3,475.3	14.1	24,604.4	194,036.2
1982	12,298.2	41.1	13,388.9	44.7	4,239.1	14.2	29,926.3	211,828.3
1984	13,431.1	40.0	15,556.7	46.3	4,589.1	13.7	33,577.0	239,757.1

Source: Accounts Division, Ministry of Health and Welfare, Health and Welfare Statistics in Japan, Tokyo, 1988

benefits, improved health insurance provisions and the introduction of free medical care for elderly people – coincided with the oil crisis and thus government plans to expand public spending came just as Japan entered a time of low as opposed to high annual economic growth; between 1955 and 1973 the economy had grown at an average rate of 10.5 per cent per annum. But the growth rate for 1970–5 was 4.7 per cent.[4]

Medical treatment and pensions still account for the major share of social security benefits; medical care benefits have however been declining as a percentage of the total – from 59 per cent in 1970 to 40 per cent in 1984, with 1975 being the first year when medical benefits dropped to less than 50 per cent of the total. Pension benefits by contrast have been increasing, growing from 24 per cent in 1970 to over 46 per cent in 1984, the shift reflecting the growing numbers of people covered by pension schemes and a series of substantial hikes in the level of benefits (see Table 5.2).[5]

In discussing health care expenditure we have to keep in mind the usual strictures about the absence of universal standards of accounting for health care or indeed for the structural components of a health care system. Japan has her own accounting systems and definitions for health and medical care and there are significant limitations to the data which are presented here on health expenditure. First, there are no all-inclusive figures on the totality of health care expenditure; our discussion is based on the official statistics on national medical care expenditure (NME), which include costs covered by health insurance, public medical care, and the sums paid by each patient for health and medical services in hospitals, clinics, and doctors' offices. These official statistics on NME do *not* provide data on such procedures as health check-ups, routine maternity care, abortions, optical services, and medical research; NME also omits costs associated with extra-charge hospital beds (private or semi-private), personal nursing care, and attendants which are a common feature of Japanese hospitals. Nor does NME describe expenditure on capital development by either the government or the private sector and this is considerable. As we saw in Chapter 1, Japan is well down the league table for health spending as a proportion of national income and yet it tops the international tables for life expectancy and infant mortality-rates.

National medical care expenditure in 1984 was 15,093.2 billion yen or 125,500 per capita: this was equivalent to 6.30 per cent of national income.[6] Japan, we can see, is therefore spending less on health care than all but a few of the developed OECD countries and considerably less than its major economic and trading partners. At first sight it stands as something of an exception to the theory that 'Countries with relatively high incomes tend to spend proportionately more of their GDP on health services than those with lower incomes'.[7] It is likely though that the theory would also hold true for Japan if a factor were added in to the NME figures to capture the additional personal spending on health care which the official statistics miss out. To do so would add some 3–4 per cent it has been calculated, and Japan's true health expenditure to GNP ratio is more correctly represented by a figure of 9–10 per cent.

In 1982 public funds from national and local governments accounted for 4,935.3 billion yen or 35.6 per cent of NME, insurance contributions for 7,437.6 billion yen or 10.8 per cent (see Table 5.3). The Ministry of Health and Welfare reported in June 1988 that national medical expenditure reached a record high of 17.07 trillion yen during the fiscal year 1986.[8] This represented a 6.6 per cent increase over 1985's figure of 16.16 trillion yen, it accounted for 6.4 per cent of national income and per capita medical costs were 140,300 yen. In issuing these latest statistics the ministry confirmed that the country had failed to achieve policy goals of holding down growth in medical expenses to a level at or below the growth in national income, which was 4.1 per cent in 1986.

In Table 5.4 we can see total annual medical care expenditure for the years 1955 to 1982. Japan has been able to keep its total NME to a low proportion of national income but it would be foolish to ignore the fact that the growth-rate each year has been a massive one. Annual percentage increases in NME reached double figures in all but two years (1956 and 1971) up until 1979 when more stringent government policies aimed at curbing health spending began to be implemented. The country was able to support this level of increase in NME thanks primarily to average annual growth in the economy in the order of 10.5 per cent between 1955 and 1973.[9] None the less annual percentage growth in NME has been consistently higher

Table 5.3 Changes in national medical expenditure (100 million yen)

	1960	1965	1970	1975	1980	1981	1982	1983	1984	1985
National medical expenditure	4,095	11,224	24,962	64,779	119,805	128,709	138,659	144,800	149,000	157,200
Public funds	804	2,911	6,901	21,709	42,545	45,540	49,353	49,600	47,800	46,000
Items Insurance contributions	2,063	6,001	13,241	34,636	63,722	68,897	74,376	78,300	83,300	91,500
Payment by patients etc.	1,229	2,312	4,820	8,435	13,538	14,271	14,929	17,000	17,900	19,600
Medical care expenditure per capita (Y1, 000)	4.4	11.4	24.1	57.9	102.3	109.2	116.8	121.2	123.9	130.0
National subsidy to medical care expenditure	642	2,478	6,031	18,825	36,464	38,996	42,146	44,100	42,100	38,900
(Rates) (Unit: 1)										
Medical care expenditure growth rate (over previous fiscal year)	13.0	19.5	20.1	20.4	9.4	7.4	7.7	4.4	2.9	5.5
National income: growth rate (over previous fiscal year)	20.4	13.8	19.7	9.9	8.6	4.7	4.1	4.3	6.0	6.2
Medical care expenditure as portion of national income	3.09	4.22	4.10	5.26	6.17	6.34	6.55	6.56	6.37	6.33
National subsidy as portion of medical care expenditure	15.7	22.1	24.2	28.9	30.4	30.3	30.4	30.5	28.3	24.7
Medical care expenditure breakdown: Public funds	19.6	25.9	27.7	33.5	35.5	35.4	35.6	34.3	32.1	29.3
Insurance contributions	50.4	53.5	53.0	53.5	53.2	53.5	53.6	54.0	55.9	58.2
Payment by patients	30.0	20.6	19.3	13.0	11.3	11.1	10.8	11.7	12.0	12.5

Source:

1 Figures shown above for Medical Care Expenditure for the years 1960–82 are based on 'Medical Care Expenditure' by the Statistics and Information Department of the Ministry of Health and Welfare; later figures are estimated from the respective annual budgets.

2 National Income figures for the years 1960 to 1983 are taken from the Economic Planning Agency analysis; later figures are taken from the report from 'Economic Prospect for FY 1985 and Basic Economic Management Policy'.

3 Population figures are as of October 1 for 1960 to 1983 as announced by the Statistics Bureau of the Prime Minister's Office. Figures for 1984 and 1985 are from the report named in Note 2.

Table 5.4 Annual national medical care expenditure (NME), Japan, 1955–82

Fiscal year	*NME* Total (1,000 million yen)	*NME* % Increase over previous year	Expenditure per capita (1,000 yen)	*Proportion of NME* To GNP %	*Proportion of NME* To NI %
1955	238.8	11.0	2.7	2.69	3.27
1956	258.3	8.2	2.9	2.60	3.16
1957	289.7	12.2	3.2	2.58	3.10
1958	323.0	11.5	3.5	2.74	3.36
1959	362.5	12.2	3.9	2.66	3.29
1960	409.5	13.0	4.4	2.53	3.09
1961	513.0	25.3	5.4	2.58	3.26
1962	613.2	19.5	6.4	2.83	3.48
1963	754.1	23.0	7.8	2.95	3.66
1964	938.9	24.5	9.7	3.17	4.01
1965	1,122.4	19.5	11.4	3.35	4.22
1966	1,300.2	15.8	13.1	3.30	4.18
1967	1,511.6	16.3	15.1	3.27	4.11
1968	1,801.6	19.2	17.8	3.29	4.18
1969	2,078.0	15.3	20.3	3.20	4.09
1970	2,496.2	20.1	24.1	3.32	4.10
1971	2,725.0	9.2	25.9	3.29	4.14
1972	3,399.4	24.7	31.6	3.53	4.38
1973	3,949.6	16.2	36.2	3.39	4.13
1974	5,378.6	36.2	48.6	3.90	4.80
1975	6,477.9	20.4	57.9	4.27	5.26
1976	7,668.4	18.4	67.8	4.50	5.54
1977	8,568.6	11.7	75.1	4.54	5.61
1978	10,004.2	16.8	86.9	4.84	6.00
1979	10,951.0	9.5	94.3	4.93	6.13
1980	11,980.5	9.4	102.3	4.97	6.17
1981	12,870.9	7.4	109.2	5.05	6.33
1982	13,865.9	7.7	116.8	5.18	6.55

Source: Statistics and Information Department, Ministry of Health and Welfare, Tokyo, 1985

Figure 5.1 Changes in national medical care expenditure by origin

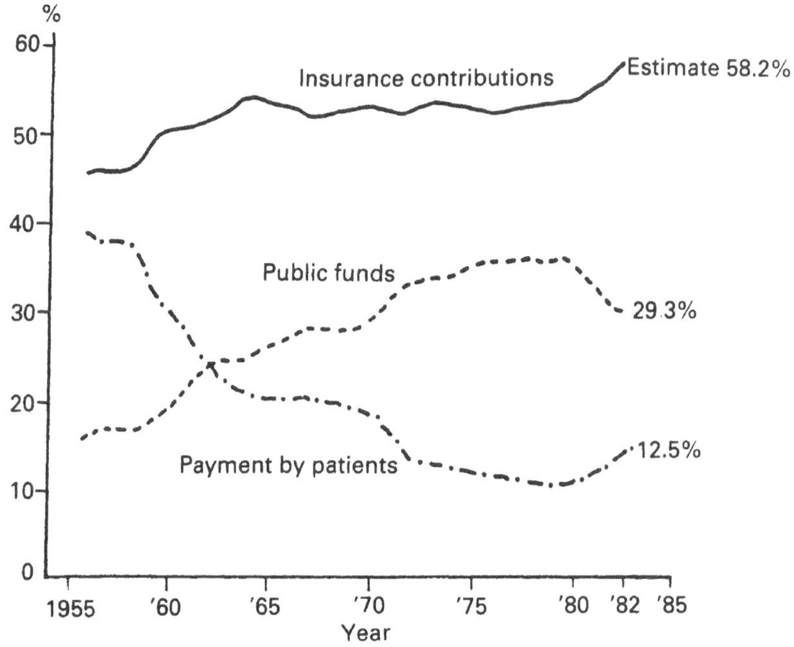

Source: 'National Medical Care Expenditure', Statistics and Information Department, Ministry of Health and Welfare Estimate based on Budget for 1983 to 1985

than the percentage growth in national income.[10] This cannot realistically be sustained.

There have been significant changes in the sources of spending over the same period, as we can see illustrated in Figure 5.1. The proportion of spending derived from public funds grew steadily until the beginning of the 1980s when government policies changed. Payments by patients – that is co-payment for services at the point of delivery – declined throughout the period, dropping especially steeply in the first half of the 1960s when universal health insurance was introduced and social welfare programmes expanded. Another sharp drop is evident after the introduction of free health care services for elderly people in 1973. The general trend through the 1960s and early 1970s of greater public funding has been noted and put into reverse by government policies for the 1980s. In the future there will be further reductions in the proportion covered by public funds and increased co-payment by patients, this being an important element in official policy to discourage excessive demand for health and medical care.

We have seen that medical care costs in Japan have risen at a faster rate than the country's economic growth. A number of factors, the same as those at work in other developed countries, have contributed to this increase. The four principal reasons have been first, demography and specifically the fact that many more people are surviving into old age than ever before, which makes greater demands on health care resources. Second, changes in patterns of disease, with chronic diseases becoming more prominent. Third, progress in medical technology and the development of new drugs and therapies. And fourth, the general public is better informed, has higher expectations about medical sciences, and is demanding larger quantities of health care. The ways in which these factors interrelate and interreact in contributing to rising health care costs vary from country to country and we shall assess how they have worked in Japan and what policy measures have been designed to counteract them.

First, population structure. Japan in common with other developed countries is experiencing the ageing of its population; more and more people are living longer and elderly people will be constituting a larger proportion of the total population. However up until the 1980s Japan's population was ageing rather more slowly than that of other developed nations: 9 per cent of the population was aged 65 and over in 1980 in Japan compared with 14.6 per cent in Britain, 15.3 per cent in West Germany, 13.8 per cent in France, and 11.0 per cent in the USA.[11] The process is now accelerating and by the beginning of the twenty-first century Japan will find itself with the highest proportion of elderly people of all the developed countries. By 2025, the year in which the proportion of elderly is expected to peak, it is estimated that they will constitute 21.8 per cent of the population (see Figure 5.2).

Ironically when other developed countries saw their health costs explode and had to evaluate the nature of their health services in the light of this new population factor, Japan's age structure would appear to have worked in her favour and helped to keep the ratio of medical care costs comparatively low. In other words had Japan had a similar proportion of elderly people in the population as other countries throughout the 1970s (e.g. West Germany) then she would have recorded a health spending to GNP ratio of 7.5 per cent rather than 6.2 per cent in 1979.[12] Nevertheless Japan is experiencing the same process as elsewhere with regard to the consumption of health and medical services by elderly people and expenditures will rise simply in order to maintain the same levels of care. Japan is no

Figure 5.2 International comparison of ageing of population

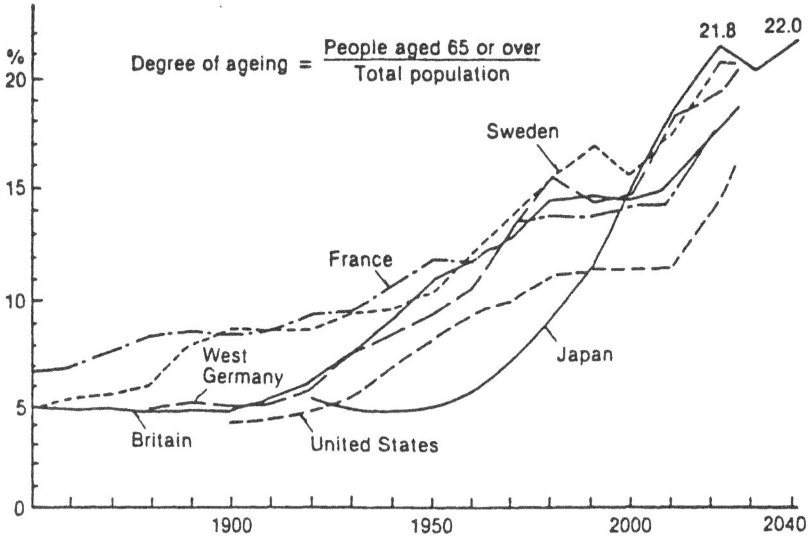

Source: Japanese national censuses: *Nihon no shorai jinko shin shikei ni tsuite* (New estimates of Japan's Future Population), Ministry of Health and Welfare, 1981; United Nations: *The Aging Population and its Economic and Social Implications*, 1956, Demographic Yearbook; *Demographic Indicators by Countries, as assessed in 1980.*

exception to the rule either that individually old people are responsible for a disproportionate share of health expenditure. The annual rate of increase in medical care costs for elderly people has been much greater than the rate of increase for the population as a whole (see Table 5.5). Other figures prepared by the National Federation of Health Insurance Societies suggest that in 1982 over one-third of medical care costs were for those aged 65 and over and that per capita the medical care costs for this age group were four times the national average per capita. Average per capita was put at 102,000 yen and average per capita for those aged 65 and over at 359,600 yen.[13] For elderly people, moreover, in-patient costs accounted for 56.3 per cent of expenditure whereas for the population as a whole in-patient costs were below 50 per cent of the total.

As part of the social welfare expansion of the 1960s and early 1970s the Law for the Welfare of the Aged of 1 January 1973 introduced free medical care for elderly people: costs of the programme were met by government and private health insurers and topped up by central government subsidies. However the many insurance schemes did not have equal numbers of elderly members: the proportion of elderly people covered by the national health

Table 5.5 Trends in national medical care costs and medical care costs for the aged

Year	*National medical care costs (100 million yen)*		*Medical care costs for the aged (100 million yen)*		*Ratio of medical care costs for the elderly per national medical care costs*
		Rate of increase (%)		*Rate of increase (%)*	
1974	53,786	36.2	6,652	55.1	12.4
1975	64,779	20.4	8,666	30.3	13.4
1976	76,684	18.4	10,780	24.4	14.1
1977	85,685	11.7	12,872	19.4	15.0
1978	100,042	16.8	15,948	23.9	15.9
1979	109,510	9.5	18,503	16.0	16.9
1980	119,805	9.4	21,269	14.9	17.8
1981	128,709	7.4	24,281	14.2	18.9
1982	138,659	7.9	27,487	13.2	19.8
1983	145,438	4.9	33,185	—	22.8
1984	150,932	3.8	36,098	8.8	23.9

Source: 'Investigation by Department of Health for the Aged', Ministry of Health and Welfare, *Outline of Social Insurance in Japan*, 1986, p. 45, Tokyo: Japan International Social Securities Association

insurance scheme was twice that in other, mostly private, health insurance schemes and the government was forced during the 1970s to subsidize a disproportionate and growing share of medical care costs. Clearly this situation was unpalatable to a government intent on reducing public spending. Furthermore the health insurance system based on fee-for-service payments tended to provide greater compensation to medical services-providers and institutions for concrete items of service with emphasis on curative rather than preventive care; such a pattern of health care is not necessarily appropriate to the needs of the elderly chronic sick. From the financial and service point of view therefore, the system needed some rethinking and a considerable overhaul. The work of various committees and study groups resulted in policy proposals which led to the Law of Health and Medical Services for the Aged of August 1982 which was implemented in January 1983. The three major features of this revised Act are: first, abolition of the earlier system of free medical care for the aged. Provision of free services was criticized because it was thought to reduce individual responsibility for health care and health awareness; old people, uninhibited by anxiety about cost, were said to be taking advantage of the free services to consult their doctors too frequently and unnecessarily. Since 1983 elderly people are required to make a co-payment at point of service. Second, the share of medical care benefits for elderly people contributed by the different insurers was modified to redistribute the cost burden more equitably among various medical insurance schemes. Finally, a number of measures were devised as a means to improve preventive health care and to enhance individual health awareness. At present it is difficult to assess the extent to which these particular recommendations have been carried out across the country as a whole.

Let us turn now to the second factor which has contributed to the increase in health expenditure – changes in patterns of disease. Chronic disease particularly cancer and diseases of the circulatory system have shown a large rise in incidence in Japan, especially in the last twenty years, and we described this in some detail in Chapter 3. These diseases are not amenable to short-term or one-off treatment procedures but rather require lengthy periods of care and therapy. In the period since the Second World War service provision in Japan has become increasingly hospital-based and the fee-reimbursement system has fostered this development. Hospitalization rates are low in Japan for all age groups except elderly people but the average length of stay is extremely long for the whole population and even longer for the elderly.[14] Alternative forms of care and facilities such as nursing homes and community services are poorly developed and hospital is the only place available. Because of the structure of the medical care system with its private, free-enterprise nature there is a lack of co-ordination and integration between the medical care services provided by individual practitioners, clinics, and hospitals and between the medical care services and the social welfare programmes which may be available through local governments. Many community services are subject to means testing and services such as home helps or home nursing (if and where they are available) are not covered by insurance benefits. The end result is that it is easier, both financially and practically, to put an aged or chronically sick relative into hospital as costs will then be met by insurance benefits.

Japan is justifiably renowned for its ready grasp of new technology and its inventiveness in electronics and computer technology. The rapid increases in the use of expensive and sophisticated diagnostic and therapeutic appliances is a third factor in contributing to the cost spiral in health care in the country. Again the free enterprise basis of the health system has contributed to this. Compared with other countries the speed with which CT (CAT – Computerized Axial Tomography) scanners, kidney dialysis equipment, and the provisions of intensive care units and other items associated with 'advanced', technological medical care have been introduced has been quite remarkable.

The smallest clinic may well be equipped with the kind of equipment which elsewhere might only rarely be available to the staff of specialist or university teaching hospitals. Such facilities have enormous value in attracting new clients to the practice and in enabling the clinic owner to proclaim himself as a specialist practitioner to the public. The medical supplies and equipment companies operate aggressive sales and marketing programmes and purchase arrangements usually involve 'options' to buy the next model in the series when it is produced. Once purchased, the equipment must be paid for. The existing point-fee system does not include reimbursement for some procedures – this is the government's method of controlling and rationing the use of new technology, an approach which is logical and effective. Thus medical practitioners and hospitals cannot pass on to the insurance companies the real cost of the extra services which they provide; they can however recoup their investment costs in other quite legitimate ways by an astute use of the point-fee system, the control mechanisms of which cannot at present effectively prevent a proportion of slippage. Individual practitioners or facilities can perform other diagnostic tests and examinations which cost less, or they can prescribe additional, perhaps not always totally necessary, medication; the net result is that sufficient total income can be made without too much difficulty and the costs of the more expensive procedures met without any undue impact on operating profits.

The fourth contributory factor to the increase in health care expenditure is public demand, which in itself has been fuelled by greater awareness about developments in medical science and technology and greater expectations about the outcome of medical care; a large expansion in the number of medical practitioners and facilities has improved access to medical services and given the public a much greater choice about the type of service they can obtain. The introduction of health insurance during the 1950s and subsequent expansion of coverage and benefits eased any potential financial burdens which may have inhibited individuals from taking advantage of the many more doctors, clinics and hospitals. The provision of free services for the aged undoubtedly caused a massive increase in the utilization of available services and facilities by this age group, beyond what might be accounted for by the sheer increase in population numbers. Although by comparison with other developed nations the hospitalization rate for Japan is low, the rate has doubled since 1960; the numbers of facilities and private medical practitioners have likewise grown dramatically. In 1950 there were 91.9 physicians per 10,000 population and by 1982 there were 141.5 per 100,000 population.[15] This growth stemmed largely from government policy for dealing with the acute shortage of doctors during the 1950s and this was to encourage and provide financial help with the development of new medical schools.

Hospitals and available beds have grown by 150 per cent in the past thirty years with most new facilities being in the private sector. In the absence of a co-ordinated service delivery system or referrals between hospitals and small clinics or individual practitioners the pattern has evolved whereby hospitals maintain a large ambulatory case-load in order to ensure a good supply of in-patients as well as income; individual practitioners too carry high patient case-loads – the so-called 'kamikaze' doctor who sees as many as one hundred patients per day is not an uncommon phenomenon – in order to keep income levels high enough. The health insurance system normally reimburses without too much elaborate checking or verifying of bills submitted. Doctors prescribe from their own pharmacy and under the existing reimbursement system can expect to make approximately 20 per cent profit – the difference between the point-fee system amount and the actual amount they pay the drug company for the drugs. Drugs account for more than one-third of total medical care costs. Using government-managed health insurance as an example it has been estimated that in 1980 drugs contributed 38.2 per cent of medical care costs and in clinics (as opposed to hospitals) the ratio is much higher – 44 per cent of total costs.[16]

The Japanese tradition of providing a large share of medical care via ambulatory service cannot be under-estimated for its significance in keeping costs down while helping to meet rising demand for services. But there has been a noticeable trend towards greater use of hospitals for all kinds of services, and this, not surprisingly, has had substantial impact on the distribution of costs.

Expenditure on in-patient services totally has increased some twenty-six times since 1962 with clinics (defined as facilities with fewer than twenty beds) now accounting for less than 10 per cent of such expenditure. In addition to providing a growing proportion of in-patient services the hospitals have also accounted for more out-patient expenditures – 36.2 per cent in 1983 compared to 28.9 per cent in 1962. The trend towards greater and hence more costly hospital-centred services and provisions is one which Japan's health care policy-makers are concerned to control and change in order to achieve cost controls in the future (see Table 5.6).

Financing health and medical services

Having seen how much Japan has spent in the post-war years on health care, and described the main factors which have influenced

Table 5.6 National medical expenditure for in-patient and out-patient services, 1962, 1975, 1983

	1962	*1975*	*1983*
Total expenditure	6,132	64,779	145,438
Hospital in-patient services	2,072	22,640	55,689
Hospital out-patient services	875	10,356	28,812
Clinic in-patient services	272	2,787	5,605
Clinic out-patient services	2,153	23,319	41,881
Dental services[a]	759	5,677	15,565
Pharmacy services[b]	NA	NA	2,882

Source: Ministry of Health and Welfare, Tokyo, 1986
Notes: [a]Expenditure on dental care includes expenditure on dental care at hospitals.
[b]Expenditure on prescribed drugs at pharmacies was estimated separately from 1976.

the total amount and patterns of health expenditure, let us now examine how the money is raised and how health and medical services are paid for.

Roemer distinguished six major health care services financing mechanisms, noting that most countries usually employ all of them but that the proportion of health care costs covered by each varies from country to country.[17] The six mechanisms are

1 personal payment by the individual to the service-providers,
2 provision of services by charitable organizations, usually at no or little cost to the individual,
3 services organized and paid for by industry,
4 private health insurance taken out by individuals on a voluntary basis,
5 social insurance covering health care, often required by law,
6 general revenue support for services, raised by local or national taxation.

The United Kingdom's National Health Service is an example of provisions which are centrally organized and funded out of government revenue and voluntary private insurance accounts for a minor part of health financing. The USA on the other hand has traditionally relied on private health insurance although in recent years there has been considerable growth in employer-financed health insurance together with a growth in government financial provisions especially to pay for services for those not covered by insurance (Medicaid and Medicare). The European countries demonstrate a wide variety of arrangements predominantly based on insurance schemes which are wide-ranging in membership base, contributions, benefits, and reimbursement mechanisms.

It will perhaps not surprise many readers to learn that Japan has a system of health care financing which appears at first sight to be marvellously straightforward, but which on further study is revealed to be a massively complex and fragmented structure. Taking the German social insurance system of the early part of the century as its model, Japan has yet again contrived to work the trick of creating something which, once foreign, has been moulded into something which is perfectly acceptable and suitable to Japan's culture, identity, and concepts of social equity, in other words something intrinsically Japanese.

Health insurance was the first form of social insurance to be introduced in Japan; enforcement of the Health Insurance Law, passed in 1922 and modelled on the German Krankenkasse, was delayed until 1927 because of the Tokyo Earthquake of 1923. The purpose of the Law was 'to provide for the payment of benefits to insured persons and to persons supported by them in case of sickness, injury or death irrespective of causes or sources, including occupational ones or maternity' (Article 1).

The legislation was introduced at a time when Japan was industrializing rapidly and undergoing great social change; it was initially aimed at providing protection for workers employed in small enterprises – some of the larger companies had earlier started to provide industrially based medical services for their workers. Total enrolment came to just under 2 million; benefits were limited, a number of diseases not included, the maximum period of payment was 180 days for the same illness and hospitalization required the approval of the insurer.[18] This was the beginning of the structure which exists today and which has been expanded incrementally and unevenly but which has not been substantially reformed. The next major improvement in the system came in 1938 with the National Health Insurance Law which introduced insurance cover for the self-employed, casual workers, farmers, fishermen, and merchant sailors; in 1940 cover was extended to non-manual employees in private organizations and some limited benefits for dependants were introduced – half the cost of medical care was paid for. Several more employment-related social insurance schemes, which included medical cover, were set up through the late 1940s and 1950s:

1947 Workmen's Compensation Insurance
1953 Day Labourer's Health Insurance
Private School Teachers and Employees Mutual Aid Association Insurance
1958 Staffs of Agriculture, Forestry and Fisheries Institutions Mutual Aid Association Insurance

The revised National Health Insurance and National Pensions Acts of 1959, enforced in 1960, represented a concerted effort to ensure universal cover for health care and pensions provisions. It was a commendable move but did not alter the essential nature of the insurance systems which have remained, until today, quite different in benefits and contribution rates. The National Health Insurance Act required local authorities to inaugurate medical insurance schemes to provide insurance cover for those individuals (residents of the authority) who were not members of an employment-related scheme. During the 1960s and 1970s further measures were taken by government to expand and upgrade the whole social insurance system: medical and pension insurance benefits were increased, workers' accident insurance was extended, a number of social welfare provisions were started, such as child allowances and public contributions schemes for old age pensions (for those not involved in company pensions plans). These many reforms did produce more or less universal medical insurance cover and this is the situation today.

The system broadly comprises two major groupings of subsystems which are first, Employee Health Insurance for employed individuals and their dependent family members, and second, National Health Insurance for self-employed individuals, farmers, retired people, and their dependants. Additionally there is the system for the aged which is an amalgam of the two.

All the schemes are similar in terms of the range of medical service covered, the procedures for obtaining medical care and the system of reimbursing medical practitioners and institutions; but there are significant differences in eligibility, administration, cost-sharing, cash benefits, financing and the level of national government subsidy provided to defray administrative costs and make up deficits. Over and above insurance there are residual programmes financed by local and national governments under the public assistance scheme which provide limited, and means-tested, assistance to the needy. National government has also assumed responsibility for the medical care and treatment of specific population groups, e.g. those with TB, specified infectious diseases, nuclear irradiation sufferers, and those with disease eligible for treatment under the Health Damage Compensation Law.

To say that there are two principal types of insurance schemes with membership based on employment status is to oversimplify the matter, as we shall see when we look at the details of the various schemes (see Figure 5.3). In *Employee Health Insurance*, an individual employed by an organization obtains health insurance cover for himself and family through membership in one of a

Figure 5.3 Number of insured persons classified by health insurance scheme, 31 March 1986

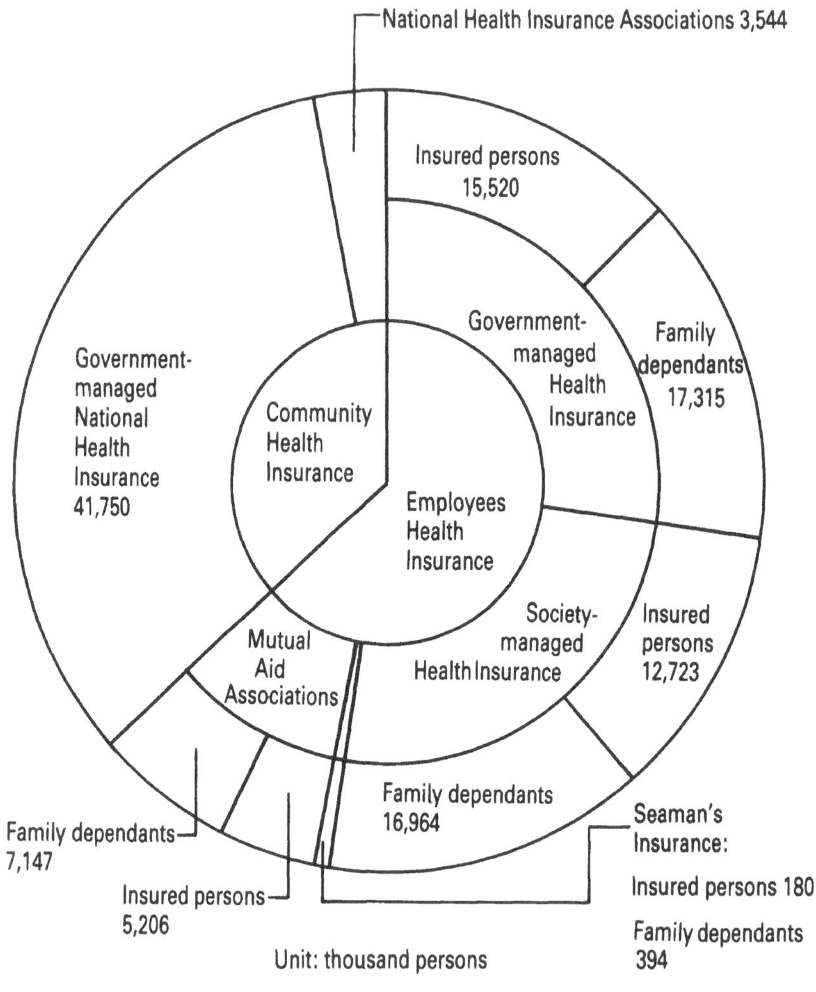

Source: Outline of Social Insurance in Japan, p. 9, 1986

number of schemes, one group of which are basically private and the other public. These are

1 Government-managed health insurance, members of which are normally employed in smaller firms whose insurance is managed by the government.

2 National government-managed schemes designed specifically for day labourers and seamen.
3 Health insurance societies cover employees of large organizations, where the insurance programme is managed by a separate corporate body. Where a company is large enough – usually with more than 300 employees – the health insurance programme will be operated purely for the employees of that organization. One or more companies can also join together to set up and manage a health insurance scheme.
4 Finally, there are three groups of mutual aid associations which run schemes for local and national government civil servants and for the teaching and other staff members of educational establishments.

The government-managed schemes in this group are distinct from the government health insurance system which is called *National Health Insurance*. This is community-based and provides cover for those people who are not included in any of the above employment schemes. Since 1984 this too has comprised two subdivisions: one for agricultural workers and self-employed people and one for the aged. National Health Insurance is administered by local governments – cities, towns, and villages. There are also the so-called National Health Insurance Associations which manage insurance for groups of individuals who may work in the same trade or profession, such as medical practitioners, and architects who are usually self-employed or classed as the owners of small businesses. Figure 5.4 shows all the insurance schemes, the size of their membership, contributions, and benefits.

Benefits and contributions

Generally speaking, individuals covered by the mutual aid associations and the society-managed insurance schemes receive better benefits than those covered by the government-managed health insurance schemes for employees. Those insured under National Health Insurance receive the least-generous benefits. There is no doubt that salaried employees with one of the large corporations such as Mitsubishi, Sony, etc. do better than their counterparts employed in a small local or family-based concern. Both groups of insurance cover the costs of an extensive (but not complete) range of medical services, such as consultations, pharmaceuticals, therapeutic appliances, surgery, hospitalization, hospital nursing, and transportation for such treatment. Preventive health care activities, such as screening or check-ups, and normal delivery expenses are not

Figure 5.4 Status of the medical insurance schemes, April 1987

Scheme			Insurer (as of March 31, 1987)	Number of Insured Per (As of March 31, 1987) Insured persons dependents Unit: 10,000 persons	Insurance benefits: Medical care benefits: Medical benefits	Insurance benefits: Medical care benefits: Dependents' medical expenses
Employees' Health Insurance	Health Insurance – Regular Employees	Government-Managed Health Insurance	National Government	3,262 [1,543 / 1,719]	90% *80% from day following Diet approval	. Inpatient 80% . Outpatient 70%
Employees' Health Insurance	Health Insurance – Regular Employees	Society-Managed Health Insurance	Health Insurance Societies 1,777	3,005 [1,302 / 1,703]		Same as above (additional benefits available)
Employees' Health Insurance	Health Insurance	Day Labourers Health Insurance	National Government	23 [15 / 8]	*Deductible will be ¥100, ¥200 or ¥800 depending on cost of medical treatment provided at desired facility, total bill not to exceed ¥3,500.	Inpatient 80% Outpatient 70% Same as above
Employees' Health Insurance		Seamen's Insurance	National Government	54 [17 / 37]		
Employees' Health Insurance	Mutual Aid Association Insurance	National Public Service MAAs Local Public Service MAAs Private School Teachers and Employees MAA	27 MAAs 54 MAAs 1 MAA	1,235 [520 / 715] (As of March 31, 1986)		Same as above (additional benefits available)
National Health Insurance		Agricultural Workers Self-employed, etc.	Cities, towns, villages 3,270 National Health Insurance Associations 167	4,529	70%	
National Health Insurance		Retirees from Employees' Insurance	Cities, Towns, Villages	National Health Insurance Associations 297 (As of March 31, 1986)	Insured person: 80% Dependents: inpatient 80% outpatient 70%	

* Health and Medical Services for the Aged (End of fiscal 1987)	[Operating entity] Head of city, town, or village	5,312 Employees Insurance 1,883 National Health Insurance 3,429	

Source: Health and Welfare Services in Japan, 1988, Ministry of Health and Welfare, Tokyo, p. 45

High-cost medical expenses	Cash benefits	Financial resources Insurance Contribution	National government subsidy for medical care benefit costs	Percentage receiving health and medical services for the aged (%) (as of March 31, 1986)
Patient maximum deductible ¥54,000 (¥30,000 for low income persons)	Injury and sickness allowance Maternity allowance Delivery expenses, etc	8.3% Special insurance contributions 1% (Since March, 1986)	16 4% of benefit costs	4 2
*Total medical expenses per household (When 2 or more payments exceeding ¥30,000 each (¥21,000 each for low income households) are made, benefits cover the total expense)	Same as above (additional benefits available)	8 103% (Average for all societies, as of March 31, 1987)	¥6,700 million as benefit cost assistance (Fiscal 1987)	2 8
	Same as above	Grade I ¥140 per day Grade II ¥1,970 per day (Since April, 1986)	16 4% of benefit costs	14 3
Abatement for households with repeated applications (Patient deductible is lowered to ¥30,000 (¥21,000 low income households) from the 4th application made in 12 months)		8 2% (Since April, 1982)	None	5 4
	Same as above (additional benefits available)	6 50–11 914% (As of March 31, 1987)	None	3 8
Abatement for patients suffering from disease requiring costly treatment (Patient deductible is ¥10,000 for hemophiliacs and those suffering from chronic insufficiency of the kidneys requiring regular dialysis)	Midwifery expenses Funeral expenses Nursing allowances, etc (Optional)	Contribution based on individual income, assets etc	50% of benefit costs 32%-52% of benefit costs	12 4
			None	

Patient cost sharing Outpatient ¥800 per month Inpatient ¥400 per day (¥300 per day maximum two months for low income persons)	Provided by each Insurer of health insurance	(Share of costs) National government 2/10 Local governments 0 5/10, 0 5/10 Insurers of each health insurance 7/10

included although a lump sum maternity allowance is paid under some schemes to cover some of the costs of normal birth.

Monthly premiums paid by the insured individual differ depending on the scheme and are usually a proportion of monthly salary, the total contribution for an employee being made up of a contribution from the employer, the employee's share being deducted from salary. The employee's share is determined by a special formula, which takes into account gross income and family size and may be less than the employer's contribution in society-managed schemes and equal in government-managed schemes. Figure 5.4 also shows details of the percentage contributions.

This monthly premium does not however take complete care of the individual's outlay for health care. Under Employee Health Insurance the insured employee is required to make a 10 per cent co-payment for any services; dependants are required to pay 20 per cent in co-payment for in-patient services and 30 per cent for out-patient treatment. Under National Health Insurance cost-sharing is higher with a flat rate 30 per cent co-payment required of both the insured and dependants. Exceptions are retired people who pay 20 per cent; their dependants are required to make the same co-payments as their counterparts in Employee Health Insurance. Under both systems there is a ceiling on the total monthly out-of-pocket expenses and above this amount the government defrays the costs as part of its 'Costly Medical Expense Benefit' scheme. Currently the ceiling is 54,000 yen per month per person; or 30,000 yen per month per person for low-income families and lower variable limits for households and individuals suffering from specified diseases which require costly long-term treatment. Under both systems cash benefits are available such as injury and sickness pay, the maternity allowance, and funeral expenses.

Examples of average annual contributions in 1982 were: under National Health Insurance 101,329 yen per household; 189,959 yen per insured person under government-managed health insurance shared 50:50 by employer and employee; and 238,650 yen per insured individual under society-managed health insurance, again shared 50:50 between employer and employee.[19]

The monthly premiums form the major part of the insurance scheme's income but Treasury grants and subsidies are also made. Again these differ between the two schemes. Subsidies to society-managed health insurance are relatively small and are related to the financial structure of each fund; the national government picks up the administrative costs of all seven schemes in this sector. The society-managed schemes have in the past operated more efficiently than the government-managed ones – the age structure and risk profile of their members and consequently income sources being such that they have been able to keep outgoings below income. Subsidies from government to all Employee Health Insurance schemes have been less than 10 per cent of expenditures. Government subsidy to the National Health Insurance on the other hand covered about 45 per cent of benefits in 1982 as well as administration costs.

The final component in this byzantine edifice is the scheme which finances Health and Welfare Services for the Aged, which has operated since 1984 and was introduced with the intention of reducing the cost share carried by the government. The scheme covers individuals aged 70 and over and disabled persons aged 65–69; it is administered by cities, towns, and villages. The programme provides the whole range of medical benefits with limited cost sharing; individuals are entitled to the same range of benefits conferred by membership of Employee Health Insurance depending on which of the schemes they belonged to prior to retirement. Medical care expenses are financed via national government contributions (20 per cent), local government (10 per cent), and all other health insurance carriers (70 per cent). The last of these is divided among the insurers to reduce the discrepancy resulting from differential membership ratios: 11.3 per cent of NHI members are elderly as compared to 2.8 per cent of society-managed health insurance members and 4.1 per cent of government-managed employee health insurance.

What happens then when an individual falls sick and seeks medical treatment and how are the services of medical practitioners and facilities paid for? Patients seeking care can attend any hospital, clinic, or practitioner's office and are required only to present their insurance membership card in order to obtain treatment or service. Practically all facilities accept any person regardless of their insurance group, although there are some indications that NHI-insured individuals may not always be so welcome by some facilities and private practitioners. Individuals make their co-payment at the time of service in the case of an out-patient visit/consultation. For in-patient care the patient will be presented with a bill for co-payment at the end of the hospital stay, having been advised in advance of the likely cost of the course of treatment. Medical facilities are reimbursed on a fee-for-service basis and the procedures are as follows. The medical facility makes up the bill for each patient, using a tariff called the Point Fee Schedule; on this schedule each item of medical treatment has an allotted number of points and the value of the point currently is 10 yen. The account for each patient is therefore calculated by multiplying the number of items of service by the point fee. Institutions and practitioners are reimbursed the calculated remuneration per patient less the standard co-payment (usually already made by the patient).

We have seen that there are a vast number of health insurance carriers – fortunately processing of bills and reimbursements have been centralized so that facilities and practitioners do not have to submit bills to each insurance organ. All the insurance carriers transfer funds to one of two semi-government bodies – the Social Insurance Medical Care Fee Payment Fund in the case of Employee Health Insurance and the Prefectural Federation of National Health Insurance Associations, which reimburse the medical care providers according to the fee schedule. The fee schedule itself is determined by the government, the Ministry of Health and Welfare, working together with the Social Insurance Medical Council, which is made up of representatives of the insurers, the medical professions (doctors, dentists, and pharmacists), and selected public interest groups. The point fee system is a continuing bone of contention between the government and the medical profession, the latter not always agreeing with the point scores assigned to certain procedures and activities and unhappy about the omission of certain procedures. One major disadvantage of the system is that consultations with doctors are reimbursed at a standard rate, that is a facility receives the same amount for a consultation with either a junior staff member or a leading expert; the reimbursement does not therefore take into account qualifications or experience as the hospital has to do in paying its physicians.

The Social Insurance Medical Care Fee Payment Fund was established in 1948 to examine medical care bills and reimburse service-providers. It has its headquarters in Tokyo and branch offices in all the prefectures and procedures are standard throughout the country. Each branch office has a staff of scrutineers who are medical practitioners, usually employed on a part-time basis. They check all bills submitted by facilities and practitioners and are authorized to question or delete unnecessary diagnostic or treatment procedures. Once all the bills for each facility are approved the total amount of reimbursement is calculated and the facility paid. The whole process usually takes about two months. The number of claims has risen dramatically as can be seen from Table 5.7: it has been estimated that each scrutineer must now check some 13,000 claims per month.[20] Consequently the process has become superficial and oriented towards merely counting the numbers of procedures. This slack monitoring process provides ample opportunity for padding of bills: instances of facilities and practitioners taking advantage of this are growing. In 1986 a leading Tokyo University Hospital was ordered to refund about 15.7 million yen to

Table 5.7 Medical insurance claims dealt with by the Social Insurance Medical Care Fee Payment Fund, 1950–83

Fiscal years	*Total for year*[a]	*Monthly average*[a]
1950	40,041	3,337
1960	162,627	13,552
1970	326,949	27,246
1980	505,352	42,113
1983	510,649	42,554

Source: Outline of Social Insurance in Japan, 1985, Japan International Social Securities Association, Tokyo, 1986
Note: [a] In thousands.

health insurance organizations, and 38.5 million yen worth of 'unnecessary' charges to patients; over a three-year period the hospital had been steadily overcharging in six departments, a quarter of the total.[21] In all approximately 1 per cent of claims are rejected, it has been estimated. This seemingly low proportion of inaccurate claims can be viewed in one of two ways: either the number of incorrect bills submitted is indeed very small or the checking procedures are inadequate and too many dishonest claims are getting through. In view of the above-mentioned incident and government plans to tighten up the system, there is some justification in concluding that the latter case is more likely. The Prefectural Federation of Health Insurance Associations is the fund's counterpart for the scrutiny and reimbursement of National Health Insurance bills; it is organized again on a prefectural basis and operates in similar fashion. Figure 5.5 illustrates the process.

The fundamental structure of health care financing in Japan will not undergo any change in the foreseeable future. The government introduced a series of measures in 1984 which point the way to future reforms in the health insurance system. The two objectives of reform are

> to maintain medical care expenditure at an adequate level now and for the future [and] to ensure a fair distribution of benefits and contributions among the various insurance schemes. The differences . . . should be levelled so that the health insurance system as a whole can continue to be treated as a social insurance institution.[22]

Specific measures to be implemented are first, rationalization of medical fees: the point-fee and fee-for-service basis of paying medical practitioners and facilities will remain as it is, but it is recognized that there is urgent need for reform of some aspects of

Figure 5.5 Flow charts of medical care insurance operations

(1) Health Insurance (Government-managed)

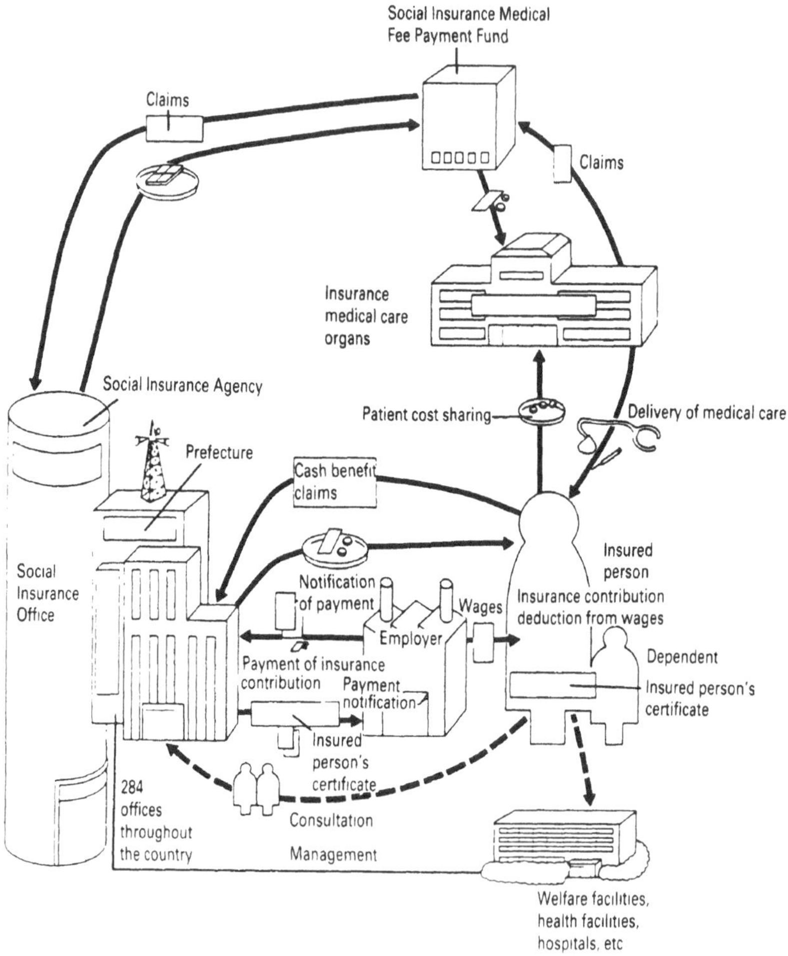

N.B. 1 In the case of Society-managed Health Insurance, the functions of the Social Insurance Agency, prefectures and social insurance offices are performed by health insurance societies

2 As of July, 1987

Source: Health and Welfare Services in Japan, 1988, Ministry of Health and Welfare, pp. 46–8

Figure 5.5 (continued)

(2) National Health Insurance

(a) National Health Insurance for ordinary person

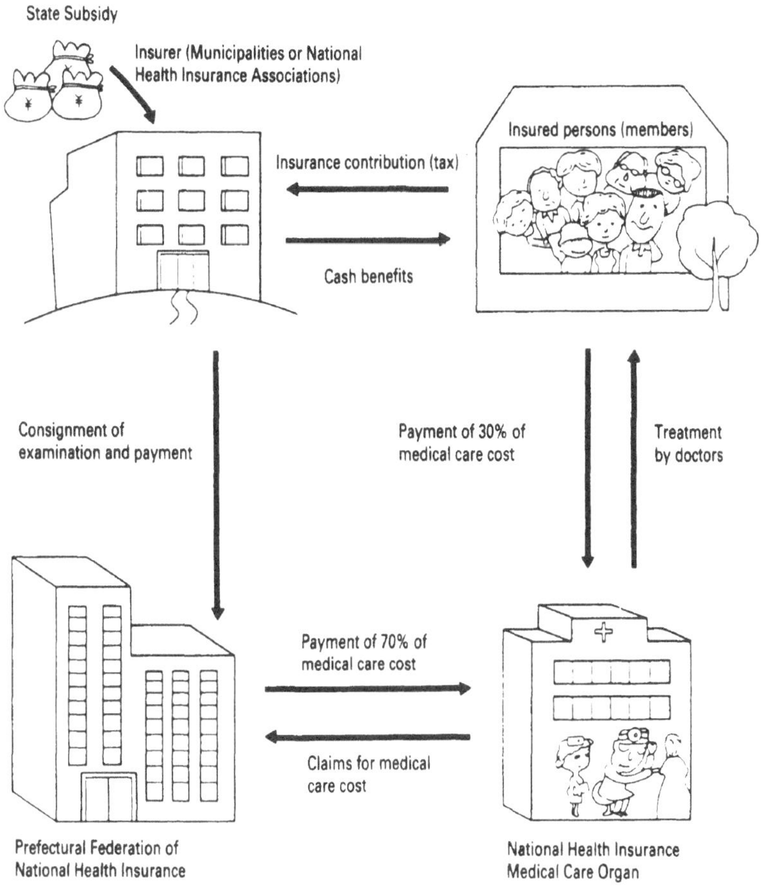

Figure 5.5 (continued)

(2) National Health Insurance

(b) Retirees' Health Insurance

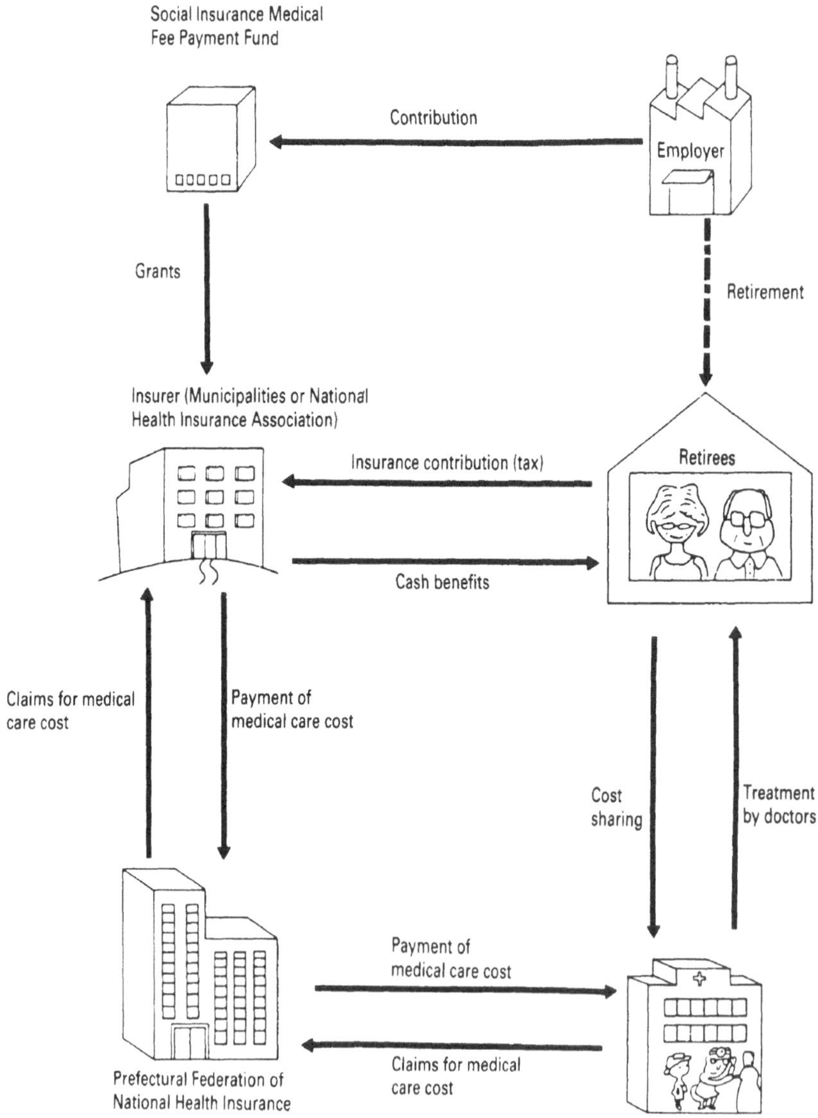

the scheme without introducing anything quite as 'radical' as the DRGs (Diagnosis Related Groups) which are used in the USA. Some streamlining and simplification of the point-fee system will therefore be undertaken with the dual objective of closing existing loopholes which make it open to abuse and fraud, and changing the existing bias towards rewarding tangible items of service. This, it is hoped, will further practitioner consciousness about the importance of delivering primary health care rather than just curative medical services. Second, work has already started and will be continued towards achieving rationalization of the tariff for drugs. Third, additional staff are to be taken on to beef up the review system operated by the Social Insurance Medical Care Fee Payment Fund in order to control abuses and cut down the numbers of excessive or illegitimate claims. Fourth, to tackle similar difficulties at the service-providers' end, monitoring and supervision of medical care facilities will be stepped up with the appointment of more supervisors and the creation of special advisory bodies. Disciplinary measures will be strengthened, including the possibility of cancellation of status as an insurance medical care facility for consistent offenders. The true impact of this lies in the threat implied by its existence rather than in its implementation. These latter two measures are aimed primarily at eliminating abuses which undoubtedly have consequences in costs to the system as a whole. Admirable though the intentions are, these reforms rather miss the point about the nature and quality of medical care; taken further the monitoring system could be used in a more positive manner to improve standards of care and professional conduct. Government proposals refer to an expansion of staff for monitoring but make no reference to the costs involved nor how they are to be covered. Fifth, differences in co-payment between the insured and their dependants and between the many insurance schemes are to be eliminated. By the 1990s it is intended that a uniform flat rate of 20 per cent co-payment at point of service will apply to every individual. Official reasoning is that users of medical care are more fully aware of the costs of such care at the time of service and that a 20 per cent co-payment is a highly acceptable level in engendering cost-consciousness. This will mean too that monthly insurance premiums can be held at the same level and this method of increasing the proportion of cost carried by individuals is more attractive, for the obvious reason that monthly obligatory outgoings from salary are not affected, a reduction in monthly disposable income being more noticeable than the possibility of co-payment at time of service, the amount of which cannot be predicted. The Japanese are conscientious savers, have a strong sense of personal responsibility, and on the whole would not be disturbed or financially troubled by having to pay a contribution. Sixth, there are the proposals for Health Care for the Aged which we have already described. Finally, establishment of the Specific Medical Care Benefit: at present a number of designated advanced technology procedures are not covered by health insurance and any associated preliminary examinations, procedures, or periods of hospitalization are likewise excluded from insurance cover. Under Specific Medical Care Benefit associated activities will be covered provided that the whole service is obtained in specially approved and designated medical care facilities – usually the university or larger specialist hospitals. This mechanism is designed to tackle the uncontrolled spread of high technology procedures while also satisfying the medical profession's concern that new and effective techniques and therapies are introduced and made available judiciously.

Our description of the main features of the health insurance system in Japan provides ample and convincing evidence that social insurance for health care can become an unwieldy, highly fragmented and complicated edifice which is expensive to administer and operate. The plurality of organizing bodies has moreover led to discrepancies in contributions and benefits. It is not surprising therefore that rationalization of this system has been the focus of government policy for health care and interestingly government is the principal instigator of such reform. Despite the unwieldiness of the present system of paying for health care, it is widely accepted by individuals at it definitely confers a number of advantages such as freedom of choice with regard to doctors and facilities; the system provides an essentially uniform standard of medical care. These outweigh the minor disadvantages of differential contributions and benefit levels. People who wish to enjoy a better class of hospital room or the attentions of a private nurse have the option to do so provided they pay for these services out of their own pocket. In this way the main health financing system ensures the provision of basic medical care to everyone. Nor have the providers of medical care – the doctors and facilities – made any massive demands for change in the organization of health care financing. Despite a history of constant quibbling over details of the existing point-fee system (the scale of reimbursements and the exclusion of certain procedures for example), the medical practitioners are happy with the benefits and freedoms associated with fee-for-service medical practice and do not seek compensation via other mechanisms. Indeed the majority of practitioners are cost-conscious and operate with a striking degree of responsibility within the wide-ranging freedoms offered. One of the important disadvantages associated with health insurance – the amount of administration, bureaucracy, and paperwork required to collect premiums, process claims, and payments still remain a problem but the centralization of the process in the Social Insurance Medical Care Fee Payment Fund has facilitated some simplification. Advances in computerization together with the introduction of a flat-rate co-payment at time of service delivery and refining of the point-fee system will ease some of the administrative burdens for service-providers in the future. It is likely too that the number of insurance societies will be reduced as mergers take place in the interests of efficiency and better management, something which is predicted for the immediate future.

The measures taken indicate that Japan's policy-makers have done a great deal to come to grips with the problems associated with an insurance-based health care financing system and have made serious efforts to put into place the necessary corrective measures. The Health Care System for the Aged and the provision of residual benefits for the high-risk and needy population groups are, within the Japanese context, fairly radical moves. Measures to control cost-generating behaviour by the medical profession and to limit the spread of new technology are in place; attempts to reduce the associated administrative and bureaucratic inefficiencies are under way.

The principal goal of cost control policy has been the reduction in the share of health expenditure carried by the public purse and the evidence is beginning to show that some success has been achieved. Reference is made to Figure 5.1 once again. It is however quite possible that the impact of some of the changes will be short term and will merely delay a situation that is inevitable, given the known changes in the demographic structure of Japan by the beginning of the next century. At the same time there are other developments taking place in the social structure and fabric of Japan and, in devising its policies for the future of health care, the government and its policy-makers do not appear to have taken them fully into account, nor has a real attempt been made to evaluate possible advantages which may arise from a more radical stab at reform.

References

1 *Measuring Health Care 1960–1983 Expenditure, Costs and Performance*, OECD Social Policy Studies 2, Paris, OECD, 1985, p. 7.

2 Ibid.

3 K. Yoshikawa, *The Maturation of the Social Security System in Japan's Rapidly Aging Population*, Tokyo, Foreign Press Centre, 1982, p. 27.

4 *Japan in the Year 2000: Preparing Japan for the Age of Internationalisation, the Aging Society and Maturity*, Long-Term

Outlook Committee, Economic Council, Economic Planning Agency, Tokyo, Japan Times Ltd, 1983, p. 11.
5 *Health and Welfare Statistics in Japan, 1987*, Tokyo, Health and Welfare Statistics Association, 1987, p. 163.
6 Ibid, p. 106.
7 J.R. Butler and M.S.B. Vaile, *Health and Health Services: An Introduction to Health Care in Britain*, London, Routledge & Kegan Paul, 1984, p. 57.
8 *Japan Times*, 12 June 1988.
9 *Japan in the Year 2000*, p. 10.
10 *Health and Welfare Statistics in Japan, 1987*, p. 106.
11 Y. Naohiro, *Perspectives on the Aging Society in Japan's Rapidly Aging Population*, Tokyo, Foreign Press Centre, 1982, p. 6.
12 *Trends and Policies of Health Services in Japan: Rationalising Medical Care Costs*, Tokyo, Japan International Corporation of Welfare Services, 1983, p. 11.
13 *Situation and Trends of Medical Insurance and Medical Supply in Japan*, 1985, National Federation of Health Insurance Societies, Appendix A 14.
14 *Trends and Policies of Health Service in Japan*, p. 13.
15 M. Hashimoto, 'Health Services in Japan', in M.W. Raffel (ed.) *Comparative Health Systems*, Philadelphia, Penn. and London, Pennsylvania State University Press, 1984, p. 364.
16 *Trends and Policies of Health Services in Japan*, p. 13.
17 M.I. Roemer, 'A global view of financing and delivery patterns', in Roemer, *Health Care Systems in World Perspective*, Ann Arbor, Mich., Administration Press, 1976, pp. 14–15.
18 J. Ohmura, 'Overview of Japanese health insurance', *Japan=Hospitals*, 2, July 1983, p. 17.
19 *Health and Welfare Statistics in Japan*, 1985, p. 144.
20 K. Kiikunii, 'Quality assurance programs in Japan', *Japan=Hospitals*, 3, July 1984, p. 30.
21 *Japan Times*, 12 June 1986.
22 *Recent Japanese Policy on Health: the Background and Measures for Reform*, Ministry of Health and Welfare, Tokyo, November 1985, p. 16.

Chapter six

The medical care delivery system

The provision of personal health care services for the general public in Japan consists of a mix of public and private efforts. As we saw in Chapter 4, responsibility for the planning and implementation of public health programmes, including community health and environmental services, rests with the government at national and provincial levels. At the national level responsibility for these programmes is vested in several bureaux of the Ministry of Health and Welfare. The provision of medical care services to individuals is largely and primarily in the hands of the private sector and the ministry, though the Health Service Bureau has an advisory role and some supervisory responsibility. This system, or more correctly, pattern of care is hospital- and clinic-based and emphasis is on the provision of curative rather than preventive measures of health care. Health care in Japan is highly fragmented and any attempt to classify it according to the standard models of health care delivery systems is difficult. At best it is possible to delineate two separate systems running in parallel to each other. Within the sector which can be described as personal medical care services there are again two channels of service delivery. There are the hospitals, public and private, which provide in-patient and out-patient services; and the clinics and offices of medical practitioners, which provide ambulatory care and also offer some limited in-patient services. Links between the two channels are not formally established and co-ordination of services is therefore almost non-existent. In this chapter we provide a detailed description and analysis of these channels of service provision; we look at the nature of the health services they provide, the benefits and advantages afforded by this pattern of service delivery, and we note the problem areas. We also examine whether this pattern of provision is adequate in Japan today and whether it is appropriate to the health care needs of the Japanese population.

Hospital services

In all countries hospitals are now a vital component in the provision of health services. The ways in which hospitals have been developed and their historic roots are tremendously varied. In Europe the long history of hospitals can be traced back to the Middle Ages when the Church established places of shelter for the sick, the destitute, and the aged. Even today when the trend is towards greater government involvement in the organization and delivery of health care, there remains a considerable range and variety in the ways that countries plan, organize, and administer the hospital services which have become the corner-stone of health care.

The first western-style hospital in Japan was set up in 1557 by a Portuguese Jesuit, Luis Almeida. There were no real advances in the development of such facilities over the next three hundred years as Japanese contact with the outside world ceased. In 1861 the Yojosho Hospital set up by the Dutch in Nagasaki was one of the first western-style facilities set up as part of the massive programme of modernization which Japan embarked on at that time, known as the Meiji Restoration.

Since that time Japan has evolved and refined her own concept of hospitalization, a concept which in the latter years of the twentieth century differs in many fundamental aspects from that now current in the western industrialized nations. Despite some obvious changes in such physical features as buildings, equipment, and facilities the underlying ethos of hospital care in Japan remains very much unchanged from what it was in the early years of the century. The provisions for hospital services today reflect characteristics of their origins; private facilities predominate and the average size of hospitals is small. Japan has one of the highest bed-to-population ratios in the world, the longest average length of stay, a maldistribution of facilities, and in some areas the sheer competition for patients has lead to some unacceptable aspects of medical care and practice.

Classification of facilities

The Medical Service Law of 1948 distinguishes between hospitals, clinics, and maternity homes.[1] Hospitals are classified into four categories – general hospitals, mental hospitals, tuberculosis hospitals, and communicable diseases hospitals. There is no designation of hospital services as 'acute' and patients with chronic illnesses are normally treated in general hospitals. Nursing homes, long-term care facilities, or special facilities have not been extensively developed: traditionally the long-term care of chronically sick, disabled, or elderly people has been a family responsibility.

In legal terms the major distinction between a hospital and a clinic is essentially one of size. Officially a medical facility with twenty beds or more, with the prescribed facilities and equipment – e.g. consulting rooms, laboratory facilities, X-ray apparatus, dispensary and meals services – is designated a hospital (Medical Services Law, Article 21). Government regulations further stipulate the ratios of doctors, nurses, and other allied health personnel. Hospitals with beds for more than one hundred patients and providing internal medicine, general surgery, obstetrics and gynaecology, ENT (ear, nose and throat), ophthalmology, laboratory and pathology facilities can be designated a 'Sogo Byoin' or general hospital.

Clinics are establishments which may or may not have in-patient beds; if a clinic does have beds the maximum permitted number is nineteen and the Medical Service Law requires that patients do not ordinarily stay in the facility for longer than forty-eight hours. Nor can these facilities describe themselves to the public as a hospital.

Any individual or body wishing to establish a private hospital must obtain permission from the prefectural government through the Prefectural Health Department; facilities must meet specific requirements for construction standards, equipment, staffing, and facilities. A midwifery home must be operated by a fully qualified and registered midwife; the Medical Service Law limits the size of these facilities to a maximum of ten beds. In 1982 there were 27,388 practising midwives in Japan, two-thirds of whom were employed in hospitals, clinics, or health centres.[2] Of the remainder, 2,533 were running their own midwifery homes, where women are admitted for normal delivery. Qualified registered doctors may set up a clinic or take up practice in a locality; once they have notified the prefectural or city health department that they have done so no further licensing procedures are required.

Establishment of national facilities is restricted under the Medical Service Law Amendment no. 159, 1962, and public facilities can be set up only with the approval of the Ministry of Health and Welfare. Development of public hospitals is financed by local or national government, using public funds; this factor has been instrumental in controlling the development of such facilities.

In essence there has been no systematized planning of hospitals and clinics in Japan. A relatively recent initiative by the central government requires prefectural governments to ensure that the development of new hospitals does not lead to an excess number of beds in each local government area. The planning techniques employed for the purpose of review are rudimentary and consist largely of the application of bed:population ratios in order to ensure that desired norms are not exceeded. However the cost of developing and financing private medical facilities is not shouldered by the government and its ability to plan effectively the location, distribution, and growth of such hospitals is consequently limited; this situation has been mutually acceptable to all parties involved in the provision of hospital services.

Development of public hospitals has been more effectively controlled. In early 1986 the national government announced its intention to reduce the numbers of national government hospitals by 30 per cent over a ten-year period.[3] Responsibility for these facilities will be transferred to either local government or the private sector and in some instances facilities will be closed down. The plan has not been welcomed by the local governments, which will have to assume the running costs, nor by the health care labour unions, which interpret the plan as a threat to existing health care provisions. In this matter Japan appears to be spearheading the reversal in the trend towards increased public (i.e. government) control and involvement in the delivery of health services.

Hospital ownership

Hospital ownership is everywhere shared between the public and private sector; the exact balance of the mixture varies from one country to another and is constantly changing. In the United Kingdom the scale of private facilities is small, with about 9 per cent of all hospital beds and 6 per cent of acute beds in private facilities.[4] In Australia in 1981 70 per cent of all hospitals were public facilities and they provided 78 per cent of available beds. A mixture of private facilities owned by a variety of companies, religious groups, philanthropic organizations, and business partnerships contributed 30 per cent of facilities and 22 per cent of all beds.[5]

In Japan the two umbrella categories of ownership, public and private, can be distinguished and within each category ownership is highly diversified. This fragmented pattern of ownership greatly limits governmental ability to influence the size and function of individual hospital units directly and the whole nature of hospital care available in a particular geographic location.

Let us look first at the government sector. In the government hospitals category we can distinguish national-level facilities and local government facilities, and in each category ownership may rest with various bodies. Local government hospitals may be run by the prefecture, or the city government. In some instances a facility is owned by local government but managed by a private contractor.

The Ministry of Health and Welfare operates a number of national hospitals, mostly specialist centres which focus on research and treatment of a particular disease or group of diseases. The National Cancer Centre in Tokyo was set up in 1962 and is the premier medical institution in the country for cancer research. It is supported in its work by nine regional centres and a network of prefectural centres. The National Cardiovascular Diseases Centre established in 1977 is another example of such a national-level facility.

It is official policy to reduce the number of national *general* hospitals; in the same plan, however, the government publishes proposals to establish three new national *specialist* medical centres – a psychiatry and neurology centre, an international medical co-operation centre, and a maternity and paediatric centre. Teaching hospitals attached to the state university medical schools come under the jurisdiction of the Ministry of Education (Monbusho). There are a number of hospitals designated as national facilities which are sponsored by former government enterprises which have been privatized, such as the Japan National Railways and the Tobacco and Salt Monopoly.

Public institutions traditionally are more highly regarded than private ones in Japan and this is true even today, with the large government, national, and metropolitan hospitals enjoying a high reputation for the services they provide. Apart from the hospitals operated by the Ministry of Health and Welfare and other quasi-government agencies a variety of public non-profit organizations contribute a large proportion of public facilities. In this category there are the Red Cross hospitals and facilities owned and operated by a total of ten different groups of social insurance associations, welfare associations, and industry- or employment-related groups.

In at least one respect the private hospitals sector resembles the public sector: ownership of private hospitals is highly fragmented among many diverse groups. This situation has its roots in the early days of modern medicine in Japan and has proved acceptable to government, service-providers, and consumers alike. As owners of private hospitals we can distinguish the following. Medical schools affiliated with private universities operate their own teaching hospitals and the hospitals attached to the prestigious private universities such as Keio in Tokyo enjoy a high reputation. A number of companies, particularly those with a large blue-collar work-force, run hospitals and clinics exclusively for company employees and their dependants. However, the numbers of such facilities are small and decreasing, as it is nowadays easier and more cost-effective to provide employees with health insurance benefits which allow them freedom of choice of hospital or clinic. Then there are facilities run by schools or insurance corporations which cater to their contributors, members of staff and their family dependants. Profit-making corporations operating chains of facilities are a minor part of the spectrum to date but this sector may grow as the opportunity to merge small privately owned and financially rocky institutions presents itself as an attractive business venture. By far the majority of private hospitals are in the hands of individuals or family groups or medical care corporations, often called medical juridical persons. This last category is a relative newcomer and one which expanded tremendously in the 1960s after amendments to the Medical Service Law in 1959. Facilities run by a medical care corporation are required to have a Board of Trustees and at least three full-time doctors on staff. Government intentions underlying the amendment to existing legislation were to foster the development of a broader more public base of ownership of hospitals. This did not in fact happen, as the new legal structure simply enabled the existing individual owners to establish foundations or trusts in order to take advantage of tax and other financial concessions available to such entities.

Subsequent revisions to the Medical Service Law (1985) have removed the requirement for minimum numbers of qualified medical staff, thus allowing owners to take advantage of the tax and other concessions without having to fulfil more stringent staffing requirements attached to larger facilities. Government control over the development of hospitals is further diminished and the proliferation of small facilities remains largely unchecked. Many private hospitals continue to be run as private family businesses. The legal controls on existing hospitals are few. The prefectural government may carry out inspection but regular inspection is not required and in fact is usually only carried out in cases of medical malpractice, or where violation of the Medical Service Law is suspected. A number of spectacular cases of fraud has caused concern for the Ministry of Health and Welfare; a special 'medifraud inspectorate' was appointed in 1983 to monitor insurance claims.

Hospital supply

In 1983 (as Table 6.1 shows) there were more than 9,000 hospitals in Japan, the majority of which (88 per cent) were classified as general hospitals. In the past thirty years the total number of medical care facilities has increased by 150 per cent, with the greatest growth being in numbers of private facilities and taking place during the 1970s, spurred on and facilitated by a combination of public demand, favourable government policies, improvements in medical insurance coverage, and the availability of a generous supply of qualified physicians.

Table 6.1 Hospitals by type and category of ownership, 1983

Ownership	*Hospital type*				
	General	*Mental*	*Leprosaria*	*TB and contagious diseases*	*Total*
National	426	3	13	—	442
Local government and other public	1,177	50	—	19	1.246
All private	6,845	951	3	28	7,827
Total	8,448	1,004	16	47	9,515

Source: Medical Care Facility Survey, Statistics and Information Department, Ministry of Health and Welfare, Tokyo, 1984

The numbers of facilities and beds continue to grow steadily and growth is unlikely to be greatly reduced, even though there may be a slowing down in developments in the private sector. Government policies for the coming twenty-five years will have real impact only on the development of national and public facilities. Between 1970 and 1983 the total number of general hospital beds grew by almost 50 per cent and has quadrupled since the end of the Second World War. The declining incidence of infectious and communicable diseases has meant that the number of specialized hospitals and beds has dropped.

We have noted that hospital ownership is highly diversified in Japan, with some twelve major sponsors of medical care facilities in the public sector and a varied range of private owners. For the sake of clarity we have restricted presentation of data to three major groupings: national, local government and other public, and all private owners. Appendix 4 lists details of all the categories of hospital owners and sponsors and shows how we have reclassified them. In 1983 the whole public sector (i.e. national, local government, and other public bodies) sponsored just under 19 per cent of all general hospitals, 5 per cent of mental hospitals, thirteen out of the sixteen leprosy hospitals, and 40 per cent of the tuberculosis and communicable diseases facilities. Private owners and organizations account for 81 per cent of all general hospitals, 95 per cent of mental hospitals, the remainder of the leprosy hospitals, and 60 per cent of the tuberculosis and contagious disease hospitals. If we consider all the medical care facilities together it is clear that the private sector is responsible for providing most (82 per cent) of all facilities; local government and other public bodies (the minority) run 13 per cent of all facilities and the national government just

Table 6.2 All hospitals and general hospitals by category of ownership, 1951–83

Ownership	*1951*		*1960*		*1970*		*1983*	
	Total	*General*	*Total*	*General*	*Total*	*General*	*Total*	*General*
National government	391 10.3%	195 6.3%	452 7.4%	238 4.8%	444 5.6%	392 5.7%	442 4.6%	426 5.0%
Local government and other public	654 17.2%	485 15.8%	1,425 23.3%	1,252 25.4%	1,388 17.4%	1,282 18.6%	1,246 13.1%	1,177 13.9%
All private	2,751 72.5%	2,388 77.8%	4,217 69.2%	3,431 69.7%	6,142 77.0%	5,195 75.6%	7,827 82.3%	6,845 81.0%
Total	3,796	3,068	6,094	4,921	7,974	6,869	9,515	8,448

Source: Survey of Medical Facilities, Statistics and Information Department, Ministry of Health and Welfare, Tokyo, 1984

under 5 per cent. In the past forty years the private sector has been the dominant one and its share of medical care facilities has grown by some 10 per cent since 1951. While national and local government facilities have grown in absolute numbers they have in fact reduced as a proportion of medical care facilities. Table 6.2 illustrates these figures.

Japan, as we have learned, developed its medical care system during the nineteenth century using the prevailing German medical system as its model; today it continues to share many similarities with the German system. Japan seems moreover to offer startling confirmation of the validity of the theories concerning the distribution and size of hospitals in a health care system which is largely unplanned and dependent on the private sector. As noted by Abel-Smith, a hospital 'system' consisting mostly of privately owned and operated facilities tends to result in the majority of the facilities being small.[6] As we can see illustrated in Figure 6.1 and Table 6.3, this is indeed so in Japan today; private sector facilities in particular are especially small units. Among hospitals with independent or private ownership the average number of beds per facility was just ninety-seven in 1983. There is evidence of a trend towards larger units and the situation today is quite different from that in 1951 when approximately 80 per cent of medical care facilities had fewer than one hundred beds; the proportion of such small facilities had dropped to 57 per cent in 1970 and declined further to 51 per cent in 1983 with most of the change taking place in the reduction in the numbers of very small facilities, that is those having fewer

Figure 6.1 Number and size of hospitals, 1951, 1965, 1975, and 1983

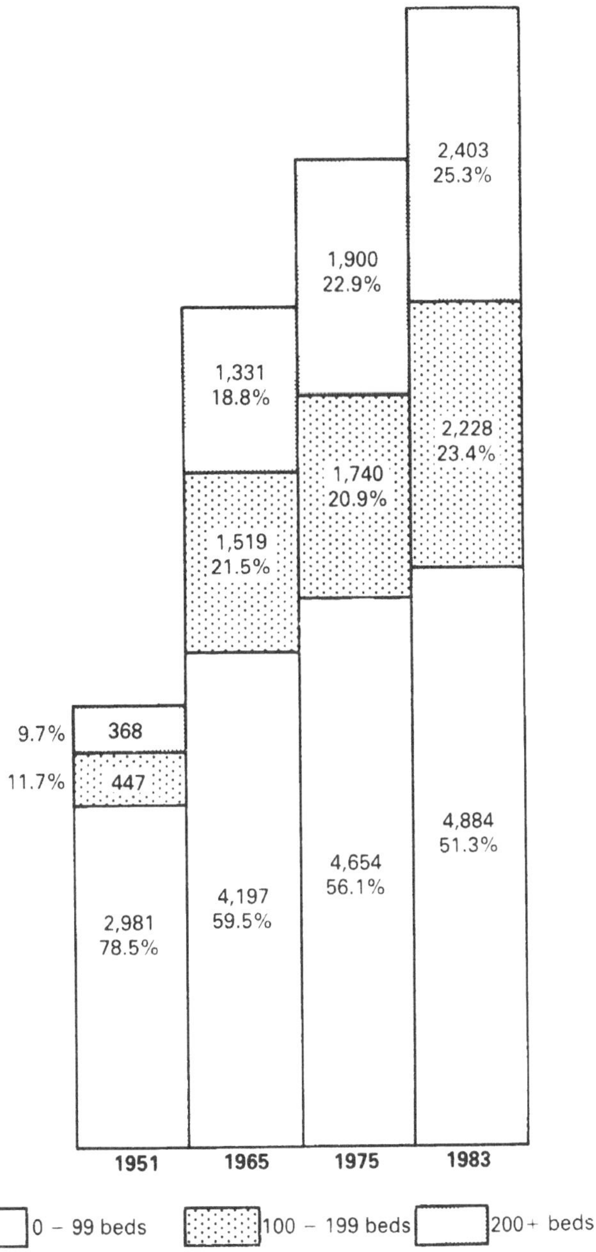

Source: Surveys of Medical Facilities, Statistics and Information Department, Ministry of Health and Welfare, Tokyo, 1986

Table 6.3 General hospitals and general beds, by ownership, 1983

Sponsorship	*Hospitals*	*Beds*	*Average number/unit*
National	425 5.0%	120,344 11.8%	282
Local government and other public	1,177 13.9%	234,295 22.9%	199
All private	6,845 81.0%	668,587 65.3%	97
Total	8,448	1,023,226	

Source: Survey of Medical Facilities, Statistics and Information Department, Ministry of Health and Welfare, Tokyo, 1984

than fifty beds, and a growth in the number of units having between fifty and one hundred beds.

The proliferation of small facilities, which are officially designated as hospitals, has grown over the years out of what were originally the clinics and surgeries of individual doctors who gradually added in-patient accommodation, developed and offered specialist services and treatment, and invested in new premises and facilities. There are a number of reasons for this pattern of growth. It was obviously more convenient for doctors to have their patients on the spot than to have to go out to the patient's home or to make arrangements for nursing care at the patient's home. At the same time the larger government and prestigious private hospitals, such as those attached to the medical schools, operated closed systems and doctors in private practice in the community had no admitting rights; doctors who referred patients to such a facility for treatment they could not provide would be *de facto* giving up the care of those patients. Many doctors were reluctant to do this and preferred to expand the range of care they provided. A more cynical interpretation is that referral of patients would also deprive doctors of income; hence the impetus for the development of in-patient accommodation by many private doctors lay rooted firmly and deeply in the medical profession's own pockets.

As we have indicated, government input in the planning of health care and the required medical facilities has been deliberately kept to the minimum; what planning it has attempted has been aimed primarily at controlling expenditure on medical care rather than at any fundamental alteration in the established private-based system set up in the nineteenth century. With the expansion of medical care insurance in the early 1960s, private clinic doctors were assured of a steady income, which grew along with public demand for medical services; funds were thus available for investment in new technology and equipment and for the expansion of premises. Some argue that the smaller hospitals and clinics today are acutely aware of market forces and consumer demands in Japan for the latest piece of technology and therefore are under considerable pressure to attract patients and keep them for the long term. The All Japan Hospital Federation, which represents the interests of private hospital owners, supports the continuation of the present hospital system and patterns of provision, provided that some care is exercised; the appropriate government policies therefore developed to prevent the willy-nilly application of new diagnostic and therapeutic technology, which has contributed to the explosion of costs of medical care in recent years. Even though such facilities may be useful in attracting customers, many of the more enlightened hospital owners are beginning to question the value of such technology in the treatment of chronic degenerative diseases and in the care of the aged who now form a large proportion of their case-load.

Just as the owners of private medical care facilities in Japan present a varied group so too do the facilities themselves offer a diverse picture. Many private hospitals are in essence nothing more than a large health centre and offer basic primary medical care which is often limited in that it is not supported or linked in any way to any community nursing and other ancillary services. Then there are the larger institutions which can properly be compared to a district general hospital in Britain; these offer a broad range of specialist treatment and will invariably have the latest in diagnostic and therapeutic equipment.

Often the in-patient accommodation and the hotel services in the smaller facilities are rather spartan and the nursing care minimal; it was the custom for patients to provide their own food and clean bedding until the 1950s. Even today nursing cover remains poor in a great many private facilities as the management (usually the owner-doctor) aims to keep nurse staffing ratios to the absolute minimum legal requirement. Patients or their families often have to hire nursing assistants or domestic helpers in order to ensure that some care is available, especially at the weekends or overnight. This causes problems for both patients and nursing staff alike, but does enable the management to hold running costs down.

The growth in the number of facilities has brought with it a similar expansion in the number of available beds, as shown in Table 6.4. In 1970 there were 580.4 general beds per 100,000 population; this ratio grew by 40 per cent up until 1983, when there were 856.4 general beds per 100,000 population. Data reviewed by the OECD confirm that Japan now has one of the highest bed ratios among OECD member countries.[7] In 1982 there were 84 persons per

Table 6.4 Growth of all beds and general beds in hospitals, 1950–83

	1950	*1960*	*1970*	*1983*
General beds in hospitals	191,836	302,495	601,978	1,023,226
All beds	313,545	686,743	1,062,553	1,440,381

Source: Survey of Medical Facilities, Statistics and Information Department, Ministry of Health and Welfare, Tokyo, 1984

hospital bed in Japan, considerably fewer than in the UK (124 persons per hospital bed), the USA (169 persons per hospital bed) and Canada (145 persons per hospital bed); only in Sweden were provisions more generous with 71 persons per hospital bed.

Within Japan this generous bed supply is not uniformly distributed through all regions and as is usually the case the urban areas enjoy better provisions than the rural ones. In the absence of any clear-cut government policy for the planning of medical care facilities each prefecture demonstrates remarkable variations both in the level and quality of medical care facilities and in the sponsorship of them.

While the number of hospital beds per 1,000 people for Japan as a whole was 118.1 in 1982, the range went from a low of 72.9 per 1,000 in Saitama Prefecture to a high of 247.3 per 1,000 in Kochi Prefecture (see the map in Appendix 1, p. 243, for the location of these regions).[8] The maldistribution of medical care facilities has resulted from a combination of geography, changes in the distribution of the population, social developments, and a lack of planning. Over the past forty years Japan has experienced first the rapid urbanization of its society and then the process of suburbanization, especially around the principal centres of Tokyo/Yokohama, and Osaka/Kyoto/Kobe. The process has been accelerating as the newly affluent salaried employees seek better living conditions by moving out of the cities themselves into commuter belts around the major industrial and commercial centres. This has caused further peculiarities in the distribution of medical care facilities and services. The formerly rural prefectures immediately adjacent to Tokyo Metropolitan area and Osaka/Kyoto have experienced very rapid population growth; Saitama Prefecture to the immediate north of Tokyo has the lowest number of beds per 1,000 population in the country; and Chiba to the east of Tokyo and Kanagawa to the west are the next most poorly provided prefectures in the country as a whole. Residents of these areas therefore rely on Tokyo hospitals for specialized services and treatment which are not available more locally. The predominant category of ownership is also different among the forty-seven prefectures. Iwate Prefecture, a mountainous and less densely populated region on the north-east coast of the main island of Honshu, has a larger number of public hospitals. Again geography and demography combined to produce conditions which were not favourable for the development of private medical care facilities and local government has had to take action to ensure that adequate provisions were developed to meet the needs of the population. Fukushima Prefecture, on the other hand, has had a more favourable environment for the successful development of private services and hence has fewer public hospitals and a preponderance of larger private units offering a comprehensive range of services.

Hospital funding and finances

The national government provides capital funds for national hospitals; capital development of public hospitals is financed by the relevant prefectural or municipal government out of tax revenues and national subsidies. Privately owned hospitals and medical facilities can draw on a number of commercial or public sources. Leading sources of finance for the development of medical care facilities are the Medical Care Facilities Financing Corporation and the Pension Welfare Service Public Corporation, both of which provide long-term loans at low interest rates. Both bodies are required to screen applications on a priority basis to ensure that government policy guidelines, particularly those concerning the number of hospitals and beds in any given prefecture or local government district, are adhered to. Private clinics and hospitals can of course draw on the usual commercial sources available to businesses – bank loans, and so forth – for the development of new premises or for upgrading of existing facilities.

Funds to cover operating expenditure for national, public, and private facilities are derived from insurance reimbursements made by the government or private insurance funds, and from charges to patients for extra services or facilities. All facilities and practitioners are required to submit detailed billing forms to the government-operated Social Insurance Medical Care Fee Payment Fund, which has its head office in Tokyo and branches in each prefecture. Here bills are verified and payment authorized in accordance with the prescribed fee schedule. The fee schedule is fixed, with each act of medical practice having a point score and the fee per patient being computed by multiplying the point score by the fixed unit cost. Table 6.5 illustrates data collected by the Ministry of Health and Welfare for public hospitals. Figure 6.2 shows the current standard fees for prescribed medical care and treatment. Figure 6.3 illustrates examples of standard fees for selected procedures. The standard medical fee is a continuing bone of contention between the Ministry of Health and

Table 6.5 Average daily bill at prefectural and municipal hospitals

In-patient			*Out-patient*		
	yen	*%*		*yen*	*%*
Hospitalization	5,021	30.2	Initial consultation	253	4.7
Meals	1,643	9.9	Revisits	516	9.5
Extra bed charges	1,422	8.5	Lab. examination	983	18.1
Lab. examination	1,596	9.6	X-ray	405	7.5
X-ray	485	2.9	Medication	2,313	42.7
Medication	741	4.5	Injection	190	3.5
Injection	3,045	18.3	Physiotherapy	55	1.0
Physiotherapy	137	0.8	Operations and treatment	198	3.6
Operation and other procedures	2,091	12.6			
Others	449	2.7	Others	498	9.2
Total	16,630		Total	5,411	

Source: Ministry of Health and Welfare, Tokyo, June 1984

Welfare and the Japan Medical Association, the major complaints revolving around the low level of reimbursement, restrictions on the use of certain drugs and technology, and the fact that the same level of payment for consultation applies to all physicians regardless of qualifications or experience.

In theory each hospital's or clinic's level of income is thus regulated by the reimbursement system operated by the government; however, there are opportunities to boost income and these may or may not be fully exploited by individual doctors, clinics, and hospitals. The rate for a shared hospital room is for example fixed but patients may prefer a single occupancy room, so-called extra-charge rooms, which offer more privacy and better facilities. The payment system also compels medical facilities to increase throughput in out-patient clinics, which are the source of their in-patients: the crowded waiting areas of almost any large city hospital are testimony to the high turnover. As the fee for each consultation is standardized there is a tendency to ensure that each consultation is kept as brief as possible in order to see more patients. While this may satisfy the management requirements for income it does little for the quality of care offered. Such out-patient services in the larger hospitals certainly are often superficial and the emphasis is on curative treatment rather than preventive care. A substantial portion of any doctor's income is derived from the prescription of drugs under the present reimbursement system. Traditionally doctors in Japan do their own prescribing and dispensing of medication. Coupled with popular expectations regarding the provision of

Figure 6.2 Standard fee schedule, April 1986

Consultation	A	B
Initial	1,950	1,600
Second & Subsequent		
At Hospital	700	390
At Clinic	740	400
After Hours Extra Charges		
10.00p.m.–6.00a.m.	700	
Public Holiday	2,000	
Home Visit		
Consultation Fee	2,500	
Travel Allowance		
2–10km	1,000/2km	
10km+	1,200/2km	
Daily Rates for Hospital Stay		
Standard Bed Charge	1,230	
Bedding	140	
Nightwear/Gown	50	
Hospital Administration Per Day	3,820	
Daily Rates for Nursing Care		
Hospital	1,180	
Clinic	880	
Additional Charges (Based on Nurse:patient Ratios)	410–740–1,280–2,910	
Intensive Care	4,000	
Meals: Daily Rates		
Basic Provisions	1,340	
Extras	440	
Special Diets	150–300	

Source: Statistics and Information Department, Ministry of Health and Welfare, Tokyo
Notes: Fee schedule distinguishes between two categories of facility. Group A is designated as more specialized with facilities and equipment for more intensive levels of care.
All figures in yen.

medication as a necessary part of the treatment process, it means that by comparison with prevailing standards and practice in other developed countries over-prescribing is the norm and is widespread. The pharmaceutical companies are known to be in cahoots with the medical profession in opposition to the government on the matter of payment for drugs; sales of pharmaceuticals to private facilities at highly favourable rates ensure a healthy income and profit for both companies and hospital owners.

Reimbursements are made to the institution for the services of staff physicians; all consultations are compensated at the same standard rate no matter whether the patient was seen by a senior member of the clinical staff or a relative junior. Salaried staff members are paid

Figure 6.3 Fees for selected procedures, April 1983

	Yen
Diagnostic Procedures	
Chest X-Ray	1,550
ECG	1,500
Laboratory Tests	
Urinalysis	550–750
Blood test	1,600
Surgical Procedures	
Appendectomy	43,000
Anaesthesia	5,000
Hernia	46,000
Haemorrhoidectomy	28,000
Tonsillectomy	4,000
Tonsillectomy & Adenoidectomy	11,000
Gastrectomy (Total)	150,000
Gastrectomy (Partial)	130,000
Cataract Extraction	36,000

Source: Statistics and Information Department, Ministry of Health and Welfare, Tokyo

by the facility in accordance with age and experience. There are a number of traditional and accepted practices which enable individual doctors (but not necessarily the facility) to increase their income over and above their official salary, for example gifts from patients during the two gift-giving seasons in Japan, (June and December), or at the end of their hospital stay.

Official government statistics for the fiscal year 1982 on national medical care expenditure (consisting of official fees paid to hospitals and clinics) amounted to 13,865,900 million yen or 117,000 yen per capita and represented a fourfold increase over the ten-year period 1972–82, when national income grew 2.8 times. Hospital in-patient care accounted for 38.3 per cent of national medical expenses in 1983, up from 34.9 per cent in 1975; if clinic in-patient services are included then in-patient care in 1983 accounted for slightly more than 42 per cent of national medical expenditure. Total out-patient services accounted for 45.2 per cent in 1983 down from 52 per cent in 1975 and dental services were 10.8 per cent of the total in 1982 up by just 1 per cent since 1972 (see Table 6.6).

Staffing of medical care facilities

The large national and public hospitals have a full-time medical director with a permanent salaried clinical staff of specialists and junior doctors. In teaching hospitals, both public and private, the

Table 6.6 National medical expenditure by type of service, 1962, 1975, and 1983

Type of service	*1962*		*1975*		*1983*	
Hospital in-patient services	2,072	33.8%	22,640	34.9%	55,689	38.3%
Hospital out-patient services	875	14.3%	10,356	16.0%	23,813	16.4%
Clinic in-patient services	272	4.4%	2,787	4.3%	5,605	3.9%
Clinic out-patient services	2,153	35.1%	23,319	36.0%	41,881	28.8%
Dental services	759	12.4%	5,677	8.8%	15,565	10.7%
Prescribed drugs dispensed at pharmacies	NA		NA		2,882	2.0%

Source: Ministry of Health and Welfare, Tokyo, 1984
Notes: All amounts in 100 million yen
Expenditure on dental care includes expenditure on dental care in hospitals.
Separate estimates on expenditure on prescribed drugs at pharmacies available since 1970

clinical staff also hold appointments with the parent university medical school or national research institute. On the whole the teaching hospitals are larger facilities, the average number of beds being 486, and they can support the full use of advanced sophisticated diagnostic and treatment equipment. These large facilities also have a full-time administrative staff under a director of administration, responsible for managing the business, hotel and housekeeping aspects of hospital operations. Financial management and accounting staff are a large group of personnel, the processing of insurance forms and bills accounting for a major proportion of management activity.

The national and public hospitals and larger private facilities normally employ a director of nursing, responsible for management of all nursing services, appointment of nursing staff, and supervision and co-ordination of nurse training activities if these are carried out in that facility.

The staff structure in the small private hospitals is as varied as the owners. Some 40 per cent of all practising physicians are owners of either clinics or hospitals; by law the manager of a medical facility must have a medical qualification. In smaller hospitals, those with fewer than one hundred beds, the doctor who is owner and operator is responsible for all aspects of the clinical work and for business management and administration. There is usually a business manager to manage the daily financial and administrative affairs but overall responsibility rests with the owner. In such smaller institutions the nursing staff are responsible directly to the physicians and the owner-doctor; it would be unusual to have a director of the nursing staff.

Most hospitals, no matter what their size, retain a close relationship with a specific medical school, usually the owner/doctor's or medical director's Alma Mater. This relationship is of key significance in matters of staffing and in areas of clinical practice. When a small hospital plans to expand its clinical staff or introduce a new clinical department the owner/doctor would more or less automatically refer back to his medical school or university to seek the advice of the senior professor or the relevant specialty professor on a suitable candidate. Japanese society emphasizes vertical relationships between superior and subordinate and this relationship holds good throughout the years. Even if former subordinates achieve considerable distinction in their field they would still defer to the individual who was at one time their superior.

This same strong vertical relationship exists between a university medical school, its teaching facility, and its graduates. Doctors often retain primary allegiance to their university clinical department many years after they have worked in various other hospitals, continuing the methods and practice they learned as students. Extending this informal yet at the same time highly structured and elaborate relationship, many universities have strong connections with groups of hospitals throughout the country. No legal relationship exists but these 'satellite' facilities will be staffed by graduates of the university or college and medical practice will bear the stamp of the teaching staff of the parent institution. There are both positive and negative spin-offs to this traditional practice; staff may for example be moved from one hospital to another within the informal group, often counter to the interests of the hospital department or individual doctor but beneficial to the strategic value of the hospital within the community. If a hospital's popularity is on the wane within the community (and its income therefore on the decline) it may be useful to import new staff members formerly attached to a prestigious facility in another part of the country. This will usually improve the hospital's standing within the community and boost business. In exploring some of the differences in management style in a Japanese hospital Ikegami notes too, 'In most prestigious hospitals the medical superintendents tend to be retired clinical professors who have the necessary prestige for co-ordinating the activities of their fellow doctors.'[9] While these kinds of practices ensure group harmony and a certain continuity of practice, it is often the case that the energies, skills, and potential contribution of younger members of the medical staff are gradually eroded and outdated modes of practice continued for much longer than would be the case elsewhere.

Admission to hospital and patient services

When illness strikes Japanese people can exercise a number of options; as is the case everywhere in the world they can simply decide to do nothing at all and hope that nature will right things eventually. Self-medication and treatment is another popular course of action and the preponderance of advertising for proprietary medicines confirms that for many individuals this approach is preferable to professional medical assistance. Traditional practitioners of Chinese medicine continue to enjoy public respect: treatment by an acupuncturist, chiropractor, or herbalist may offer considerable relief from pain and discomfort. The services of these practitioners are not normally included under the health insurance programmes and individuals must pay the cost of such visits themselves. Some local government health programmes help the aged with referrals to traditional practitioners and in such instances the cost of treatment will be billed to the local health department. If the decision is made to seek professional medical advice, people can visit doctors practising in their own clinic or hospital or people can choose the out-patient departments of large hospitals which function for the most part as general clinics. Under the present insurance system in Japan, people wishing to receive medical care are free to go to any facility or doctor and by simply presenting their insurance card will receive care and treatment. Insurance cards are issued to the insured and to family members who are included as the beneficiary's dependants. In principle all medical care facilities participate in the health insurance programme and the patient is not therefore deterred or prevented from seeking treatment on the grounds of cost.

Given that open access and freedom of choice are assured how then do people set about seeing a doctor? How do they choose the 'right one'? Many people rely on the recommendations of family and friends or opt for the most convenient facility in their neighbourhood or close to the work-place. General public knowledge and recognition of the most prestigious facilities – the large metropolitan hospitals, teaching hospitals, and large private hospitals – ensure that they remain popular and many people will discount the extra travel time and inconvenience in order to attend such a facility. The billboards of every suburban railway station carry a generous amount of advertising of medical facilities and for those in a hurry the convenience of a small hospital close by, usually offering the latest in equipment and technology, will be the deciding factor.

Attendance at the out-patients' department of a large hospital does not require referral nor do these departments operate appointment systems. So, prospective patients may simply turn up there and will be seen – eventually! A waiting time of between one and three hours is not uncommon for a consultation with whichever staff doctor is on duty. If patients wish to see a particular doctor they may have to wait longer or even make a return visit if that doctor is not on duty at the time. An introduction or referral by a physician to a doctor of some standing can be arranged and may well be facilitated by calling in advance and the offer of a small gift. The out-patient clinics in the larger facilities function therefore as the gatekeepers for the hospital in-patient services. Undeniably the Japanese consumer enjoys some advantages, which are intrinsic features of such an open-access system; and until recently the consumer has been content on the whole to accept some of the disadvantages associated with it. But there are signs of some consumer dissatisfaction with the present system and some hospitals are introducing staggered appointments in out-patient clinics in order to shorten waiting times. In face of increased use and demand for costly hospital services the government is encouraging clinic doctors to modify their practice and take on the role of family physician; such practitioners would have a more generalized practice than is now the case and would treat patients who currently resort to hospital out-patients for what are in essence primary health care services.

In-patient admission to a hospital is arranged by the doctor who sees the patient at the out-patient clinic; occasionally patients may be referred for admission from a private doctor who has assessed that more specialized care is required, but the decision to admit rests with the receiving facility. Officially there are no waiting lists for admission to Japanese hospitals and statistics on waiting lists or waiting times for admission are not routinely collected by the Ministry of Health and Welfare. As we have seen there is a vast range of hospitals which offer equally varied facilities and services. Demand from the public affects the larger facilities the most and immediate admission is not the norm. Depending on the size of the clinical department and its bed allocation, the relative seniority of the doctor in charge of the case, and the severity of the problem, admission may or may not be speeded up. If a delay seems likely or if patients would like a second opinion they can simply go off to another hospital and try again there. This is not uncommon and, while it keeps the patient happier, it is a clear waste of resources as the same initial consultation and any necessary diagnostic tests are duplicated and paid for twice. Under the present system very little can be done to monitor let alone control this kind of duplication of service.

Once admitted the patient is usually accommodated in a shared ward of six to eight beds. In many of the smaller hospitals the provision of basic services is not always guaranteed: patients know that it is wise to provide their own soap and towels and that it is often necessary to hire a private nurse. At the same time the standard of nursing care offered in all facilities is likely to be very good and is rated as such by the public, even though the number of nursing staff is often inadequate and Japanese nurses work under considerable pressure.

Extra-charge beds are available in many facilities and usually offer greater privacy and more amenities. Bureau of Insurance data suggest that there were just under 12,000 such beds in July 1983, by far the largest number (6,737) in the hospitals attached to the private medical schools. There are standard extra-charge bed fees reimbursed under the insurance system; but the actual amount charged by the facility may be higher than this and the patient must pay the difference. In small provincial towns the highest extra charge for a private bed in a public facility could be in the order of 5,000 yen per day. It is not unknown, particularly in the larger urban centres such as Tokyo or Osaka and especially in the more prestigious facilities such as those run by the private universities, for extra-charge beds to cost between 20,000 and 50,000 yen per day. As we can see illustrated in Figure 6.2 the standard reimbursable fee per day of 1,230 yen leaves the patient paying a substantial amount for 'extra' facilities, which often in fact do not amount to a very great deal. In addition therefore to their insurance contribution and co-payment, patients are also liable for further fairly large out-of-pocket expenses for institutional medical care. The private health insurance business has started to develop and market insurance packages designed to cover these kinds of extras.

We have made the point that Japan has evolved its own particular system of health care; a look at some of the standard indicators used to measure hospital activity will confirm that hospital care in Japan is indeed quite unlike that found elsewhere. That public demand for hospital services has increased is evident from statistics on the total numbers treated as in- and out-patients in Japanese facilities; absolute numbers of in- and out-patients have doubled since 1960 and the proportion of the population admitted has likewise more than doubled in the last twenty-five years according to surveys conducted by the Ministry of Health and Welfare. These data are illustrated in Table 6.7.

By international standards however, a very small proportion of the Japanese population is hospitalized in any year. OECD data show 6.7 per cent for Japan in 1983 compared with 11.8 per cent for France and 19.2 per cent for Sweden in the same year.[10] This low rate of hospitalization is accounted for partly by the nature of the

Table 6.7 Number of patients per day by type of medical institution, 1960, 1970, 1983

	1960	*1970*	*1983*
Hospitals			
In-patients	546	853	1,217
Out-patients	754	1,223	1,601
Total	1,300	2,076	2,818
Clinics			
In-patients	63	119	161
Out-patients	2,421	3,949	4,563
Total	2,484	4,068	4,724
Dental Clinics	705	1,104	1,331
Total			
In-patients	609	972	1,378
Out-patients	3,880	6,276	7,495
Total	4,489	7,248	8,873

Source: 'Report on Private Survey', Statistics and Information Department, Ministry of Health and Welfare, Tokyo, 1984
Note: Number of patients is the estimated number of patients who received medical treatment on the day of the survey, in thousands.

health care system itself: the large number of small clinics is such that ambulatory care predominates. The health insurance system and the structure of the fee scale further enhances this situation. Hospital out-patient departments are crowded and have a very high patient throughput; it is from these departments that many facilities derive a major proportion of their total income.

As we saw earlier Japan also has a very generous supply of beds; it would have been logical to have forecast a high rate of hospitalization as it is usually the case that high provision levels lead to high and increasing levels of use. A study of acute hospital services in London and elsewhere has confirmed the overall validity of this supposition.[11] The low rate of hospital admission in Japan therefore appears puzzling. The decision to admit patients into hospital is based on a number of factors: the nature and gravity of the patient's illness and whether it can be controlled or treated only in a hospital; the availability of a bed within the hospital; the personal and social circumstances of the patient; the availability or lack of community health care resources and support services. Hospitals may have clearly stated policies on admission of non-emergency cases and this policy will be determined by the number of beds, staffing, and operating theatres.

Historically the preference in Japan among both the public and the medical profession has been for the provision of care on an ambulatory basis and this has been a key element in the nature of the development of hospital services. Once inside the hospital Japanese patients' experience will again differ from that of their counterparts elsewhere. The length of time a patient stays in hospital is determined by several key factors. There are wide variations in length of stay in hospital from country to country, within each country from region to region, and even within one hospital from one clinical department to another. Despite the continuation of such differences there has at the same time been a universal trend towards a reduction in hospital length of stay. The considerable changes in hospital services, treatment, and care have been prompted by the development and availability of new technology and procedures for the diagnosis and treatment of various conditions; financial considerations and a greater emphasis on the more efficient use of costly resources have contributed to a reduced length of stay; the development of community resources; patient preference is often to complete the recovery at home once it has been established that their condition no longer requires specialized treatment, facilities, and nursing care.

There are of course differences in compilation of data on health services use, which make it necessary to exercise caution when making comparisons among different countries and their modes of practice. The Japanese health system does not formally differentiate between acute hospital care and long-term care; geriatric patients are usually cared for in a general hospital and their longer length of stay clearly has an impact on the total average length of stay figures for such facilities. Clinical practice and the point-fee system too make a critical impact on the average length of stay figures in Japan. Even allowing for imperfections in data and peculiarities of the system, it is impossible not to be struck by the fact that Japan recorded the longest average length of stay in the world in 1983 (49.1 days). This was down from 55.1 days recorded for the previous year but extraordinarily long when compared to other OECD countries. Japan's Ministry of Health and Welfare compiles data for type of institution and these are shown in Table 6.8. If we turn to data on specific disease entities, where we should logically expect the differences between countries to be less dramatic, Japan continues to stand out above other OECD countries. Indeed while the average length of stay for all disease categories has certainly decreased in Japan, there are some diseases for which the average length of stay has gone up (see Table 6.9).

The most important factors contributing to this are the structure of the health care system itself and traditions of medical care and practice. The hospital doctor in charge of a patient generally has full responsibility for that patient's care and progress until after

Table 6.8 Annual average hospital length of stay and occupancy rate by bed category, selected years

Bed Category	*Annual average length of stay (days)*				*Occupancy rate (%)*			
	1965	*1970*	*1980*	*1983*	*1960*	*1970*	*1980*	*1983*
Psychiatric	434	455	535	536	108.0	104.3	102.4	102.8
Communicable diseases	18	18	18	18	16.6	6.1	2.0	1.7
Tuberculosis	409	385	253	221	75.4	66.2	55.4	56.0
Leprosy	11,733	11,099	7,251	5,987	75.3	68.3	68.1	71.5
General	30	32	38	39	80.6	80.3	81.4	82.2
Average	57	55	56	55				

Source: Health and Welfare Statistics in Japan, 1985, Ministry of Health and Welfare, Health and Welfare Statistics Association, Tokyo, 1986

Table 6.9 Average in-patients' length of stay by disease and injury (day) 1970–84

	Disease and injury	*1970*	*1980*	*1983*	*1984*
I	Infections and parasitic diseases (001–139)	204.2	117.6	58.1	47.5
II	Neoplasms (140–239)	46.7	51.7	51.4	53.2
III	Endocrine, nutritional and metabolic diseases (240–279)	63.1	51.9	51.4	61.1
IV	Diseases of the blood and blood-forming organs (280–289)	51.8	41.7	41.6	42.7
V	Mental disorders (290–319)	287.5	333.3	308.8	305.4
VI	Diseases of the nervous system and sense organs (320–389)	78.3	86.4	44.0	45.6
VII	Diseases of the circulatory system (390–459)	70.6	100.4	82.7	84.2
VIII	Diseases of the respiratory system (460–519)	24.0	25.6	27.4	23.4
IX	Diseases of the digestive system (520–579)	28.3	32.6	31.4	33.0
X	Diseases of the genito-urinary system (580–629)	37.8	31.0	30.8	25.4
XI	Complications of pregnancy, childbirth and puerperium (630–676)	8.6	8.7	8.8	10.2
XII	Diseases of the skin (680–709)	24.0	22.6	20.6	21.9
XIII	Diseases of the musculo-skeletal system (710–739)	65.7	72.6	61.9	71.4
XIV	Congenital anomalies (740–759)	35.1	37.7	29.6	33.9
XV	Certain conditions in perinatal period (760–779)	19.2	12.5	15.2	12.7
XVI	Symptoms, signs and ill-defined conditions (780–799)	21.4	17.5	15.8	16.4
XVII	Injury and poisoning (800–999)	36.6	37.5	38.0	37.2
	Average all diseases	50.1	55.1	49.1	40.9

Source: Patient Survey, Statistics and Information Department, Ministry of Health and Welfare, Tokyo, 1985

completion of treatment in the hospital; it is therefore often more convenient for both patient and doctor to keep the patient in the hospital until full health and mobility are definitely assured. The lack of a referral system and a fully developed general practitioner network means that the hospital doctor must also monitor and supervise progress after discharge from the hospital. Community health care services are poorly developed in most communities and where they do exist there are no systems of liaison and communication between hospital and the government health department. The financing of hospital services offers no particular incentive to either the doctor in charge or the hospital management to speed up discharge of patients. On the contrary the present point-fee system which reimburses hospitals at a standard rate per day seems designed actively to encourage hospitals to keep patients rather longer than is medically necessary or justified. Extra days at the end of the inpatient stay cost the hospital less as the patient requires less intensive nursing care, only the basic hotel services, and treatment costs are normally decreasing. From the point of view of both patients and their families there are practical advantages associated with keeping the patient in hospital. Cramped living conditions, lack of community nursing, and other community services make it difficult to care properly for a convalescent patient. As the costs of the stay in hospital are for the most part not borne by the patient but by the insurance carriers there is no financial pressure on the family to have the patient discharged. In sum the present system seems to suit everybody concerned.

Ambulatory care

The hospital is a relative newcomer in the range of medical care provisions in Japan although, as has been the case elsewhere, there has been a trend towards greater use of hospitals for the delivery of health care and treatment and this accelerated during the 1960s and 1970s. Those patients who do not want to attend a hospital outpatient clinic, rely on self-medication, or go to a traditional practitioner have another course open to them: the small private practitioner clinics both with and without beds, which have historically made a major contribution to medical care services and continue to do so today.

In 1983 just under 300,000 (16 per cent) of all available beds were provided by general clinics (see Table 6.10), although this number represented a considerable decline in the proportion of such beds in 1960, when 24 per cent of beds were in small clinics. These figures confirm the trend, already noted, towards the development of larger

Table 6.10 General clinics, general clinic beds, and dental clinics, 1951–83

	1951	*1960*	*1970*	*1983*
General clinics	45,675	59,008	68,997	78,991
General clinic beds	86,710	165,161	249,646	285,832
Dental clinics	22,582	27,020	29,911	43,115

Source: Ministry of Health and Welfare, Tokyo, 1984
Note: Not all general clinics have beds.

general hospitals and are indicative too of some changes which are beginning to take place in the prevailing philosophy of primary medical care in Japan in the 1980s. Many former general clinics have been reclassified, simply because the addition of extra in-patient beds and support facilities has edged them out of the general clinic category into the hospital category. The greater number of general clinics do not in fact offer in-patient services at all but are in essence private practitioners' offices.

As with hospitals, the distribution and location of clinics is not uniform throughout the country; general clinics numbered 78,991, or 66.1 per 100,000 population for the country as a whole in 1983. At first glance the national average of 150.6 physicians per 100,000 population in 1982 is also generous but again there are important regional variations and provisions are often inadequate. Tokyo had 201.6 doctors per 100,000, whereas Saitama Prefecture had 86.4 per 100,000 the lowest rate for the whole country. Dental clinics have grown in number by 72 per cent since 1951; there were 43,115 dental clinics, 36.1 per 100,000 population in 1983. With 56.1 dentists per 100,000 population in 1984 the government target of 50 dentists per 100,000 population by 1985 had already been achieved.[12]

There are several aspects of primary medical care which remain problematic. The private practitioner is not a general practitioner and does not normally provide the kind of primary health care which might be comparable to that provided by general practitioners in the United Kingdom or family physicians in the USA. Japanese medical practitioners are distinguishable from their colleagues elsewhere in the world by a number of features.

Differences in undergraduate education and training are one such aspect; most doctors who elect to take up private practice do so as quasi-specialists having started to concentrate on a particular speciality at the end of undergraduate training, although by comparison with specialists in other countries their training does not have the same depth. Thus some private practitioners may be primarily paediatricians and the largest proportion of their clientele children, but they will also offer general medical care. The degree and depth of specialization is not as widespread as in the USA but it is a matter of prestige for many doctors to classify themselves as specialists rather than general practitioners. At the same time many doctors who are well established in a community are *de facto* family physicians, with a role remarkably similar to that of the general practitioner in the United Kingdom. Practitioners of this kind are in the minority and are more likely to be found in rural communities than in the big cities, where population size allows for a multiplicity of levels and kinds of doctors.

Single-handed practice is the norm and private practitioners do not have access to hospital beds or facilities for their patients. There are a number of clinical consequences of this pattern of provision. Rather like the hospitals individual doctors are often pressured into offering the very latest technology and equipment in order to attract and keep patients. As a result they may fall into financial difficulties, because loans obtained to purchase equipment have to be repaid; a steady and preferably growing income has to be assured and the only ways of doing this are to increase the number of patients in total and the number of services provided per capita. Patient throughput is stepped up – some practitioners see as many as one hundred people per day – diagnostic tests and prescriptions are increased. Over time many doctors who work in this fashion find it difficult to keep up with professional developments and their 'specialist' practice becomes out of date.

As so many doctors work on their own it is difficult too to share opinions and discuss professional matters with their fellow practitioners on the kind of regular and informal basis which is most helpful in daily work. Standards of practice, professional competence, and patient care are not monitored or evaluated by any authority and practitioners are accountable only to themselves, and of course to their patients who can, and do, vote with their feet. In view of the changing patterns of disease this relatively specialized and highly expensive pattern of service delivery is finally being called into question by some members of the medical profession and consumers too. As we saw in Chapter 4 government policy calls for greater distinction in the role and services offered by hospitals and private practitioners and stresses the provision of primary health care by the latter. The policy has yet to receive the wholehearted endorsement of the Japan Medical Association which considers it difficult to accomplish the changes required; the association still represents the following stance: 'Medical specialists also do not fully understand the idea of comprehensive primary health care and often fail to respect the person as a whole person operating in a complex social and economic environment'.[13]

The fee-reimbursement system reinforces both cultural attitudes and what have come to be regarded as traditional practices; the mechanistic approach to health care is reflected in the volume of diagnostic tests and the over-prescription of medication. Blatant practice of the latter has given rise to a popular expression 'kusuri zuke' (literally 'pickling with drugs').

Like hospital out-patients departments, private practitioners rarely operate an appointment system and patients must often endure a long wait for a brief consultation, at the end of which they will depart clutching a fistful of pills and very little idea about the exact nature of their illness. The doctor–patient relationship in Japan is one of trust. Wordless communication, so-called 'belly talk' (hara gei), is a distinctive feature of personal communications in Japan and is aided by the intrinsic ambiguities of the Japanese language. Doctors tend to explain away the problem in soothing terms without necessarily providing precise information about what exactly the problem is. For the patient to ask for this information directly might be seen as questioning the doctor's knowledge, authority and judgement. To ask too many questions is as likely to bring about a rebuttal or even a refusal to carry on the consultation. Difficulties of this kind are not unknown in other countries of course, but the medical profession in Japan remains more entrenched in its views than is the case elsewhere.

> They have never learned that talking with the patient is an important part of treatment. They do feel a pang of guilt at the time, but in the end they hide behind the excuse that this sort of thing isn't part of their duties as a doctor.[14]

Greater consumer awareness and changes in social and cultural behaviour patterns are having some impact on public views of the medical profession and the number of malpractice suits, while small, is growing. Opinion surveys suggest that the public is concerned about misdiagnosis, surgical errors, unnecessary treatment, and excessive numbers of tests.[15]

Emergency medical services

We have examined the two major components in Japan's medical care services and will now look at one final sector of the medical care delivery system. As we have seen, hospitals and clinics in Japan are autonomous self-contained facilities which operate for the most part independently of one another and of any central co-ordinating body. As in other sectors of Japanese business and industry doctors working in clinics have a relatively long average working week; a 1980 survey of physicians in one prefecture suggested that a seven-and-a-half-hour day for just under six days a week was the norm.[16] Each hospital or clinic can determine its own opening hours and that is indeed the standard practice; most hospitals do not have an accident and emergency unit and cannot provide twenty-four-hour emergency cover. It is said too that it is a brave parent indeed who would trouble the family paediatrician with a call about a sick child after office hours. Provisions for emergencies and for basic medical care in rural or remote areas of the country have been a constant concern for the government and for health care planners, who are aware of the deficiencies in the existing system. A number of measures have been enacted to ensure that some basic services are available and can be relied on. The nature of the medical care delivery system however does make it difficult to ensure any uniformity of service and standards with the result that there are considerable variations in service according to the location. Even in the cities which have generous doctor:population ratios it is not unknown for districts to be doctorless after clinic hours at the weekends. There are typical horror stories of ambulances driving from hospital to hospital with an accident or emergency case in vain search of either an open hospital or one which will actually take the victim in.

Between 1952 and the early 1970s a number of measures were implemented by the government to develop minimum emergency care provisions under the Emergency Hospitals Ministerial Ordinance.[17] From 1967 this provided for an emergency medical service centre for every 1 million people; and from 1973 one public hospital was to be designated to handle road traffic accidents in those areas where the incidence of such accidents was known to be high. In the early 1970s arrangements were made to provide subsidies for the development of communication systems between hospitals and doctors providing holiday and night-time emergency cover.

Despite these various actions on the part of the government, emergency care remained poorly co-ordinated and often patchy or non-existent in many areas as co-operation between the participating service-providers was poor. In July 1976 therefore the government established the Emergency Medical Care Working Party to review existing provisions and make recommendations to improve the system. Its proposals were made public in 1977 and the system of emergency care (illustrated in Figure 6.4) has been gradually implemented.

Fire departments operate a telephone emergency aid system and ambulances are efficient at getting to patients speedily, often under

Figure 6.4 Emergency medical service system

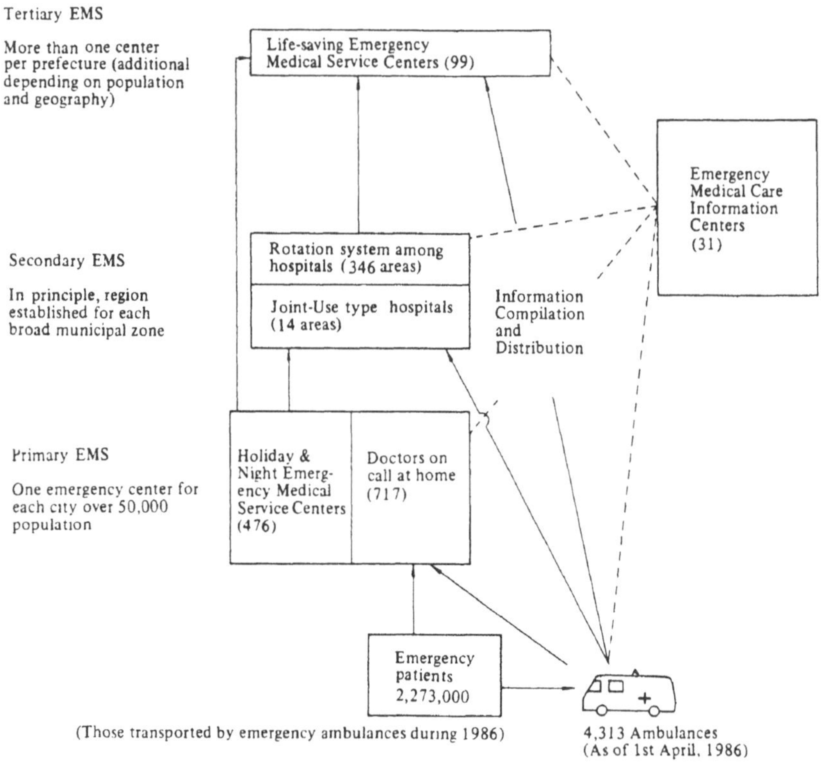

Source: Health and Welfare Services in Japan, 1988, Ministry of Health and Welfare, Tokyo

difficult traffic conditions, especially in the larger cities. Ambulance attendants are trained to provide only first aid: when they reach a patient they determine what help might be required and then attempt to obtain details of suitable hospitals and available space from the Emergency Medical Care Information Centre. Ambulances are not equipped nor their crews trained to handle women in labour and have been known to refuse to take them.

Several five- and ten-year plans have been implemented in order to ensure that medical care services are available in mountainous areas, outlying islands, and rural areas where transportation and communications may be difficult. These plans have focused on the establishment of clinics, mobile clinics, and means of transportation of patients to central medical care facilities and of doctors out to remote areas. The fifth such plan ran from 1980 to 1985 and made provisions to maintain what are known as 'Remote Area Central Hospitals', to set up health guidance offices staffed by nurses and to introduce a medical information system. Guaranteeing an adequate supply of doctors in remote areas is far more problematic. Under the present health financing system there is little incentive to private practitioners to set up practice in remote or sparsely populated districts, so outside the larger metropolitan centres doctors tend to be clustered in the smaller towns and cities. The government does offer incentives in the form of education loans for those students who intend to take up practice in remote areas on completion of their training, but a totally satisfactory solution to this problem remains to be found.

References

1 Medical Service Law (Law no. 205, 30 July 1948).

2 *Statistical Data on Nursing Services in Japan*, Nursing Division, Health Policy Bureau, Ministry of Health and Welfare, Tokyo, 1984, p. 5.

3 *Japan Times*, 10 January 1986.

4 *Social Trends 15*, ch. 7: 'Health and Personal Social Services', London, HMSO, 1985, p. 103.

5 J. Dewdney, 'Health services in Australia', in M.W. Raffel (ed.) *Comparative Health Systems*, Philadelphia, Penn. and London, Pennsylvania State University Press, 1984, p. 11.

6 B. Abel-Smith, *Value for Money in the Health Services*, London, Heinemann Educational Books, 1976, p. 101.

7 *Measuring Health Care 1960–1983: Expenditure, Costs and Performance*, OECD Policy Studies 2, Paris, OECD, 1985, p. 15.

8 *Health and Welfare Statistics in Japan 1987*, Tokyo, Health and Welfare Statistics Association, 1987.

9 N. Ikegami, 'The Japanese health system – another success story?', *Hospital and Health Services Review*, November 1984, pp. 261–4.

10 *Measuring Health Care*, OECD, p.15.

11 London Health Planning Consortium, *Acute Hospital Services in London*, London, HMSO, 1979.

12 *Japan Times*, 11 December 1985.

13 M. Yamamoto, 'Primary health care and health education in Japan', *Social Science and Medicine*, 17, 19, 1983, pp. 1419–31.

14 H. Wagatsuma, 'The right to know: A posthumous plea', in *Japan Echo*, XII, 4, 1985, pp. 70–4.

15 Nikkei High Tech Report, 9 December 1985, Nikkei Industry Research Institute, Tokyo.

16 J. Katabami, I. Kaneko, S. Oda, and M. Mugitani, 'A survey of physician activities', *Bulletin of the Institute of Public Health*, 30, 1, 1981, pp. 27–39.

17 F. Ohtani, *Medical and Public Health Services in Japan*, Proceedings of the First Asian Seminar on Health and Medical Sociology, Japanese Society of Health and Medical Sociology, 1981, p. 116.

Chapter seven

The health 'industries'

In describing the health industries of Japan we consider four specific areas. First, there are the medical service facilities, the hospitals, clinics, and other facilities which provide services direct to the general public. These were discussed in detail in Chapter 4. Second, there is the pharmaceutical industry which we describe in this chapter. Third, there are the health care equipment and medical engineering industries. Finally, we have grouped together several health-care-related service industries and a number of existing but rapidly changing health care and medical industries which are thriving in the country today: these offer impressive growth potential for the future.

We shall start by looking at Japan's pharmaceutical industry which, like so many of her multi-million dollar industrial sectors, had small beginnings and was largely derived from foreign roots.

The pharmaceutical industry

Japan's total pharmaceutical production in 1983 was 4,032.1 billion yen; with a value of just under 17 billion dollars this made Japan the world's second largest market for drug sales and consumption. Total drug production increased eightfold between 1961 and 1975, growth slowed during the 1970s but there was still a twofold increase in production between 1975 and the early 1980s. Table 7.1 shows that prescription drugs accounted for 85.3 per cent of total production and over the counter (OTC) products for 14.7 per cent. In 1983 there were 2,116 manufacturing facilities, although more than 50 per cent of total production was accounted for by a relatively small group, about a dozen, of the largest companies.[1] Antibiotics accounted for 18.3 per cent of total production in 1983, followed by cardiovascular drugs (12.6 per cent), central nervous system drugs (9.8 per cent), metabolism agents (9.0 per cent), and gastro-intestinal drugs (8.4 per cent).

Table 7.1 Monetary value of prescribed and OTC drugs, 1983 and 1984

	Monetary value of production (million yen)		*Difference*		*Proportion*	
	1983	*1984*		*%*	*1983*	*1984*
Total	4,032,057	4,026,985	−5,072[a]	−0.1	100	100
Prescribed medicines	3,438,567	3,429,482	−9,085	−0.3	85.3	85.2
Domestic production	2,382,616	2,450,987	68,371	2.9	59.1	60.9
Imported	1,055,950	978,495	−77,455	−7.3	26.2	24.3
Non-prescribed	593,490	597,503	4,013	0.7	14.7	14.8
Sold at chemists	554,738	555,759	2,021	0.4	13.8	13.8
Delivered[b]	38,752	40,744	1,992	5.1	1.0	1.0

Source: Survey of Pharmaceutical Industry Production, Pharmaceutical Affairs Bureau, Ministry of Health and Welfare, Tokyo, 1985

Notes: [a] This is the first year that production declined from the previous year since compilation of these statistics commenced in 1952.

[b] Toyama Prefecture has a system of home delivery of drugs by travelling salesmen.

In 1984 as Table 7.1 shows, less than a quarter of domestic drug consumption was contributed by imported products. Japan's pharmaceutical industry, which has grown from nothing since the Second World War, is now a mature and sophisticated industry which until recently sustained a high level of profitability on the domestic market alone. Exports have been far less important, contributing slightly more than 3 per cent of total production in 1983. But developments in the home market – the result of government measures to reduce health care expenditure – are forcing the country's leading drug companies to explore seriously the international market to expand sales and to ensure the funding base necessary to continue the research and development of new drugs and to recoup the costs already incurred in the development, testing, and production of existing inventory.

There have been substantial changes in the production, marketing, and consumption of drugs in Japan; a combination of traditional medicine practice, public expectations, and officially sanctioned research and development financing helped make the pharmaceutical industry one of Japan's most profitable and rapidly growing industries during the 1960s and 1970s. Since the beginning of the 1980s conditions once favourable to expansion have changed.

In Chinese medicine (kanpo) it was the usual practice for doctors to prepare their own compound of herbal remedies for the patient and the fee covered the costs of ingredients as well as the consultation. With the official endorsement of western medicine in the Meiji period western drugs were introduced into the country. The government issued the first Pharmacopoeia of Japan in 1886 and the profession of pharmacy became established. However, some aspects of traditional practice did not disappear entirely and doctors practising western medicine retained the right to prescribe and dispense medication from their own pharmacy. The division of responsibilities between the medical profession and pharmacists remained for a long time less clear-cut than elsewhere.

For some time after the introduction of western medical practice Japan relied almost exclusively on imported drugs, which came mostly from Germany. In the First World War imports were disrupted and the domestic industry grew in both size and quality. The industry was destroyed as a result of the Second World War but gradually started to build up again during the 1950s, relying initially on imports and developing the capability to undertake licensed production of American and European products. With assistance from the government in the form of incentives and subsidies, the industry took on a prosperity it had known in the inter-war years: production grew massively between 1961 and the mid-1970s.

Government economic policies in the post-war years were designed to encourage the growth of a number of key industries and the pharmaceutical industry was one which benefited from numerous government measures aimed at boosting the domestic market and at ensuring that the infant industry was relatively protected from the dangers of outside competition. The role played by the health care delivery system, and particularly its finance mechanisms, undoubtedly aided the sale and consumption of pharmaceuticals in the country. With the introduction of universal health insurance in 1961 demand for health and medical care was guaranteed to grow; the prevailing pattern of medical practice was such that growth in services was automatically accompanied by growth in the dispensing of medication.

The right of doctors both to prescribe and to dispense drugs, which had always enabled doctors and medical facilities to earn a large proportion of their operating funds and profits, was furthermore enhanced by the introduction of third-party payment. Doctors obtain drugs at heavily discounted prices, dispense them to their patients, and receive reimbursement of the drug's list price from the insurance funds. The point-fee system reimburses concrete items of service, such as drugs and diagnostic tests, at a disproportionately higher value than the indefinable elements of medical care and consultation. Consequently the greater the number of drugs dispensed, or injections given and tests performed, the greater the practitioner's income. With few mechanisms in the system to monitor such services individual practitioners and facilities alike have been able to take advantage of opportunities to increase, quite legitimately, their income levels. The point-fee system first of all rewards the prescription itself; second and perhaps more importantly the independence and autonomy of hospitals and doctors enables them to negotiate directly with drug companies for their pharmaceutical and other supplies. Knowing both the list price and the cost price they are well able to determine their likely profit margin on any transaction. It is often argued that control of drug costs within total health care expenditure could be more readily achieved if doctors knew more about the relative merits, demerits, and price differential between brand name products and generic products; they could consequently be encouraged or even required to prescribe the cheaper version of the same medication. In Japan doctors have long enjoyed this knowledge but have rather exploited it for their own ends; in doing so they have ignored the impact of their practice on the totality of health care costs. At one time the point-fee system was structured so that new products received preferential rates of payment to give manufacturers the incentive to invest in research and development and an added inducement to promote the use of new drugs by the doctors. The difference between the list price and the purchase price has been in the order of 10–20 per cent but in some instances was as much as 40 per cent.[2]

In prescribing a plethora of drugs at the end of a consultation the Japanese doctor is helping to meet patient expectations. In addition to prescription drugs the Japanese also have a liking for over-the-counter (OTC) preparations – vitamins, stamina pills, and stomach remedies are particularly popular; while preparations to relieve stress are also growing in significance. Doses for all medication are lower in Japan than elsewhere for reasons of safety; however, there is a tendency for doctors to prescribe longer courses of medication than their counterparts in other countries.

By the beginning of the 1980s government concern about the health care cost explosion resulted, as we have already learned, in the introduction of strict cost containment policies. Pharmaceuticals contributed more than 35 per cent of total health care costs in 1984: increases in drug prices have benefited the doctors and pharmaceutical companies, with the government footing most of the bill. The government targeted the drug tariff standard as one of the priority items for reform. The overall thrust of government measures has been to reduce the gap between government rates of reimbursement and the wholesale price of drugs. The government first therefore standardized prices on all brands of prescription medicine and then revised the formula for the point-fee system. Since 1983 procedures have been implemented to review standard drug prices every three years across the board and to carry out partial reviews each year.

The net result of these actions has been to pare standard drug prices by 35 per cent in less than four years. The government's actions succeeded, obviously perhaps, in antagonizing both the medical profession and the pharmaceutical industry, which had enjoyed a mutually rewarding relationship with each other. Now that the medical care providers are receiving lower reimbursements, they are demanding lower wholesale prices. Needless to say the once cosy relationship between the profession and the industry is now under some strain. The reforms have shown up already in static growth in the major drug companies' sales figures. Government policy is to continue to bring down the total cost of drugs within the national medical expenditure (NME) so the companies are being forced to rethink their strategy for the future. Medical practitioners too are being compelled to assess their largesse with medication as stricter monitoring of insurance claim forms is introduced in order to clamp down on excessive or over-prescribing.

With the relaxation of import restrictions and regulation the Japanese drug companies are also starting to face more competition from the multi-national pharmaceuticals companies which have for many years been anxious to enter and obtain a larger share of what has certainly been a highly lucrative market. The tight regulations on licensing and approval of pharmaceutical products in force in Japan have undoubtedly restrained the activities of foreign companies. The Pharmaceutical Affairs Bureau of the Ministry of Health and Welfare enforces a voluminous and complex body of regulations covering the manufacture, testing, approval, and marketing of drugs, quasi-drugs, cosmetics, medical devices, and other noxious or deleterious substances. The thalidomide disaster and Japan's own débâcle with SMON (see p. 185) induced the ministry to establish stricter regulations for the testing and screening of all drugs prior to licensing them for use. The first series of comprehensive regulations was introduced in 1967. Any company wishing to manufacture or import drugs must have a permit from the ministry for each place of manufacture, and approval for each item manufactured or imported.[3] The research and development of a new drug is a lengthy and costly business anywhere in the world; in Japan it is more so as requirements for test data have increased or been added to. Approval for a new drug is tightly controlled: until 1985 foreign test data were not accepted at all and any company wishing to introduce a product developed elsewhere in the world had to undertake costly duplicative testing procedures in Japan. The ministry has relaxed its requirements slightly in recent years and clinical data for tests which are unaffected by race are now acceptable. None the less drug companies are still required to carry out other additional tests in Japan in order to obtain a licence either to import or to produce locally. All drugs are also subject to re-evaluation and re-investigation, in theory every six years.

The task of screening and evaluating data is the responsibility of the New Drug Screening Committee, composed of fifteen academicians of various disciplines within the medical and pharmacological sciences. This is a volunteer body which meets approximately twice a month and is required to scrutinize and evaluate test data submitted by applicants. When submissions run to several thousand pages of documentation and data it is clear that the process cannot be a speedy one. The system forces the sponsor, the drug company, to take every possible step to ensure that investigations have been thorough and properly documented, that data are accurate and analyses correct. They must do so without specific guidelines as to the minimum requirements. The committee does not conduct hearings in order to question manufacturers on the submission or to obtain further data which may be available even if not included in the submission. Instead the company is advised of the committee's opinion and of any requirements for further information or data. If approval is contingent on the supply of further data or additional tests the company must prepare a new submission which includes the required additional information, thus in effect the whole process starts all over again. A Japanese company wishing to produce and/or sell a foreign product must prepare similarly detailed submissions; even if it has been licensed for use in several other countries it is still subjected to the same procedures as a new drug in Japan.

It has been estimated that the cost of developing and introducing a new drug in Japan is in the order of $20 million and that it takes more than a decade to get the product from the research stage into use by the medical profession; for every single product that is approved, nine others will fail the exhaustive testing procedures which are an intrinsic part of the approval procedures.

In addition to a strict system for the licensing and approval of all new drugs the Ministry of Health and Welfare has operated a monitoring system whereby designated hospitals and clinics (1,005 in 1985) and pharmacies (2,733 in 1985) are required to submit detailed reports on side-effects. Manufacturers must also submit annual assessments on all newly approved drugs until the year in which they come up for reinvestigation and an extension of their licence. Companies which discover any previously unknown and potentially harmful side-effects are required to report to the ministry within thirty days. Reports are reviewed by the Central Pharmaceutical

Affairs Council which has the authority to order revisions in both professional and consumer information about side-effects in both and recommendations about dosages and duration of use. In the worst cases manufacture and use of the product can be halted. Drug manufacturers are now required to pay a levy to the Adverse Drug Reaction Fund which was created in 1979 in order to cover provision of limited compensation and benefits (medical care expenses and invalidity pensions to individuals who have suffered as a result of taking drugs). The system is a complex one and decisions on the claim are arrived at only after a lengthy review process. Japan is not a litigious society and the preference is to settle disputes without resort to the law; in the first four years of the fund's operation 147 cases were awarded compensation.

As we have said, the world-wide disaster of thalidomide had its impact in Japan and prompted a tightening-up of procedures for drug licensing and approval. However, it was Japan's own singular contribution to the annals of iatrogenic disease - SMON - which provided the impetus for the establishment of the Adverse Drug Reaction Fund. The rationale for establishing the fund, officially at least, was to ensure protection for consumers, but the bitterness and cost - both financial and in detrimental publicity - to the drug companies and a keen awareness to avoid a repetition of the problem were the more decisive and influential factors behind the government move. The existence of the fund exercises a slightly deterrent effect on individuals who might be bold enough to take on the economic might of the manufacturers alone, that is without some official endorsement. So while the fund purports to work on behalf of aggrieved citizens it also serves to act as a buffer protecting the manufacturers.

SMON disease

The term SMON - sub-acute myelo-optico neuropathy - is essentially a descriptive term for all the features of this new disease which first began to appear sporadically in the country in the mid-1950s. The number of cases increased slowly at first but then grew quite dramatically by the end of the 1960s, eventually involving more than 11,000 cases and 500 deaths.[4] The disease ultimately affected the spinal cord, puerperal nerves, and optical nerves - patients experienced numbness and tingling in the arms and legs, muscular weakness, and in some cases blindness ensued. Most cases were preceded by diarrhoea and abdominal pain. Discovery and confirmation of the aetiology of the disease was in itself a controversial issue. It was first thought to be caused by a viral infection; others advanced the theory that it was a Japanese form of multiple sclerosis. After newspaper reports in 1969 suggested that public health experts believed it to be an infectious disease there were a number of suicides among sufferers, which served to heighten the controversy surrounding the issue. The government had set up an SMON investigation commission in 1969 to study the epidemiology of the disease and it was eventually determined that it was caused by the toxic effects of the drug chinoform (Iodochlor-hydroxyquin), a drug prescribed for stomach and intestinal upset, and especially, as time went on, for cases of traveller's dysentery. The Ministry of Health and Welfare prohibited the sale of the drug in September 1970; in the face of continuing debate and competing theories about the disease the commission continued its investigations and issued a final report in March 1972, concluding that chinoform was indeed the culprit. Cases of the disease were not common outside Japan and researchers pointed to the high dosages of the drug administered in Japan, where stomach disorders are one of the most frequent complaints and reasons for visiting clinics and hospitals. Once the drug was withdrawn, incidence of the disease fell dramatically. Proceedings against both the manufacturers and government were initiated in 1971 and by October 1984 there had been 6,436 cases at the courts. The largest hearing involved a group of 2,000 claimants in Tokyo and this reached a mediated settlement in 1977. In 1978, with a judgment handed down by the Kanazawa District Court, the claimants got the ruling they wanted, namely that Chinoform was a necessary factor in causing SMON and that the government and the drug companies had been negligent in allowing its use. Thereafter it was agreed between the state, the companies, and the patients' groups to aim to finalize all claims by amicable settlement; by October 1984 97 per cent of all cases had been so resolved.

Medical technology

Public criticism of the pharmaceutical industry became widespread at the beginning of the 1970s, largely because of the seemingly irresponsible and reckless behaviour of many drug companies. The true contribution of drugs to improvements in health care was beginning to be treated with some scepticism and the role of drugs in the medical technology revolution was taken over by a new hero, the medical engineering industry, which was beginning to apply the newly developing technology of electronics and computerization to the medical and health care field. The range and safety of surgical procedures had advanced remarkably in the post-war years; improvements in anaesthesia, aseptic and other related techniques, and the development of equipment such as the pump oxygenator, meant that many formerly high-risk procedures were now routine forms of medical treatment. As with the pharmaceutical industry advances in medical technology and engineering over the past two decades, what has been dubbed by the Japanese 'The Second Medical Technology Revolution' were fuelled by the need to keep up with medical and scientific achievements elsewhere in the world. At the same time government health care financing was critically important – expansion of medical care insurance furthered public demand for services. Equally important was official commitment and concrete support for a prosperous national industry, which was starting to feel the impact of international competition for its consumer products. In this situation it made economic sense to turn to a 'new' domestic market using and subsequently refining and improving on breakthrough technology developed in other countries. The growth of the medical engineering industries in Japan has been helped by several other factors. First, patterns of morbidity and mortality have changed and infectious diseases have been replaced by chronic degenerative diseases as the leading causes of disability and death. Second, the nature of the Japanese health care delivery system and its emphasis on the provision of concrete services encouraged the spread of multi-phasis health testing (requiring the use of complex technology and equipment) for the early detection of diseases and the subsequent monitoring and care of patients: even if the equipment could not cure at least it could confirm the doctor's diagnosis. Third, the essentially entrepreneurial basis of the health care system and its lack of government controls over the disposition of services and resources enabled individual facilities to offer some new services which might not necessarily contribute effectively to overall patient care but probably did attract new patients and therefore income. Solutions for improving and systematizing the present poorly organized emergency care services have increasingly been sought in the introduction of computerization and data communication techniques.

While a growing reliance on medical technology in day-to-day health care has been particularly striking in the past decade, the application of engineering in the medical field can be traced back further. Studies to improve the measurement of body electricity and development of the techniques of EEG (electro-encephalography) and ECG (electro-cardiography) started in the late 1940s. Japanese researchers studied the application of electrical engineering to medicine in the early 1950s; an inter-disciplinary society for medical and engineering specialists who wished to focus on research into the electro-cardiograph had already been organized in 1948. This subsequently became the Japanese Medical Engineering Society in 1962 and plays a leading role in medical engineering research and development today. The first centralized clinical laboratory for the country was established at Tokyo University in 1955. The automated blood chemistry analyser (first sold in the USA in 1957) furthered the continuation of automizing clinical lab tests in the country when facilities were opened in three of Japan's hospitals in 1960. By 1975 21 per cent of all hospitals had their own equipment. Diagnostic and therapeutic radiology has grown into one of the most capital-intensive areas in medical care. X-ray television for example which produced clearer pictures and offered greater protection for physicians and radiographers against accidental exposure to radiation appeared on the American and European scenes in the early 1950s, was introduced to Japan in the early 1960s, and rapidly grew in use through the 1970s. By 1975 60 per cent of all general hospitals and 9 per cent of private physicians' offices possessed their own equipment.

CT scanners

The introduction and distribution of CT scanners into the country probably offers the perfect illustration of how the essential nature of the health care system and government policies have worked in unity to support the dynamic growth of one industrial sector. The CT brain scanner was invented by the British electronics company EMI in 1970 and Acta Company developed the whole body scanner in the USA. In August 1975 the first CT scanner in Japan was installed in the Tokyo Women's Medical College Hospital. In the same year the Ministry of Finance ordered the import of a further thirty-seven scanners, a move aimed at easing existing Anglo-Japanese trade friction. Initially lagging behind Europe and North America in the use of the CT scanner Japan rapidly went on to overtake other countries and by 1982 had the highest number of CT scanners per million population of any country in the world (see Table 7.2). Since the mid-1970s CT scanners have been developed and manufactured in several countries. In Japan the first domestic model was produced by Hitachi-Medico; it was joined by Toshiba Medical, which in 1979 started to sell its own product instead of imported EMI models. Since the end of the 1970s Japanese manufacturers have dominated the domestic CT market with a 70 per cent share of all CT sales. Patterns of use of CT scanners differ considerably in Japan from that found elsewhere. The techniques and instrumentation of CT scanning are divided into either head or whole body scanning and when first introduced, head scanners were the most widely used. In Japan head

Table 7.2 International comparison of installed CT scanners, 31 March 1978 and 31 December 1982

Country	March 1978		December 1982	
	No.	Per 1 million population	No.	Per 1 million population
Japan	292	2.6	2,120	18.5
USA	933	4.4	2,318	10.7
UK	52	0.9	115	2.1
W. Germany	93	1.5	230	5.4
France	12	0.2	80	1.5
Sweden	13	1.6	—	—
Italy	—	—	90	1.6
Holland	—	—	80	5.7
Canada	—	—	72	3.1

Source: E. Jonsson *et al.*, 'CT Scanner Race: United States declared winner or loser', *New England Journal of Medicine*, 1978, 299: 655; O. Hasuike, 'Sharp increase in installed CT scanners – utilization is important apart from the number', *Nikkei Medical*, March 1983, 12: 208

scanners continue to comprise the majority (60 per cent of all CT scanners in use) whereas body scanners are more widely used in the rest of the world. The main reason for this difference is thought to be in differences in disease prevalence, Japan having a higher prevalence of cerebro-vascular disease.

In Europe and the USA governments have exercised various financial or other measures to control the diffusion and use of CT scanners, which are extremely expensive and require sufficient properly trained personnel to be used properly. In Japan on the other hand the government let market forces rule and purchase of a CT scanner was very much left to the discretion of individual facilities. The first generation of CT scanners was very costly but their appeal to hospitals and even small clinics was considerable. They offered a 'revolutionary' contribution to diagnostic techniques, were a strong selling-point in promoting the facility, and therefore offered conclusive proof of modernity and up-to-date medical practice. As with the purchase of drugs and pharmaceutical supplies it is up to each individual facility to negotiate the appropriate price with the manufacturer and in the case of CTs Japanese companies quickly came to dominate the market. Standard purchase agreements usually included not only maintenance and after-sales service but also some kind of option or purchase renewal clause some years hence, thus guaranteeing that the company would have a market for the newest models which it would inevitably develop within a couple of years. When CT scanners were new the government's medical fee reimbursement scheme also brought in a generous fee (30,000–60,000 yen): hospitals could be confident that they would not only meet the operating costs of the new service but also eventually make sufficient money to recoup some of their initial investment. There is no doubt that the assured income derived from government sources provided an incentive to individual facility owners. Competition soon stepped up and companies started to lower prices and develop more complex sales, service, and repurchase agreements in order to keep the orders coming in. The Japanese manufacturers also refined the product and made it more compact; prices dropped and a wider range of health care facilities were able to buy the newest CT scanner. The price of a CT head scanner – some $400,000 to $600,000 in the late 1970s – dropped to an average of $120,000 by the 1980s. Body scanners, always more expensive, have also dropped in price and they are now below $400,000. As the number of CT scanners in use mushroomed so did the cost to the government of providing the tests; it was official concern about exploding medical care costs which forced the government to review the role and utility of this particular diagnostic tool. In something of an about-turn it has started to reduce the reimbursable fee for CT tests. Initially high when the machinery was new to the country and Japanese companies were hotly pursuing the development of a domestic version, the fee has been pulled down by 30–40 per cent and individual health care facilities are being forced to adopt a more prudent attitude to the acquisition and use of CT scanners. In the second half of the 1980s, sales of CT scanners have levelled off and expansion capacity is considered limited. It is however worth noting that the phenomenal growth in the medical engineering industry during the years 1977–80 was due in no small measure to CT sales (see Figure 7.1).

CT scanners accounted for one-third of all medical X-ray apparatus sales in 1980 and 14 per cent of total medical engineering equipment. By reducing fees and thus lowering potential income for the service, the government aims to control the further growth of CT technology in the country. Total CT costs were a relatively low percentage of total national medical expenditure for example but grew from an estimated $33 million in 1978 to $137 million in 1982. The next generation of diagnostic imaging techniques, ultrasound, and magnetic resonance imaging are also being used more widely and in some instances replacing CT scanning, but use of this technology is more controlled.

Artificial organs

In the therapeutic area the development of artificial organs has

Figure 7.1 Historical trend of medical equipment sales

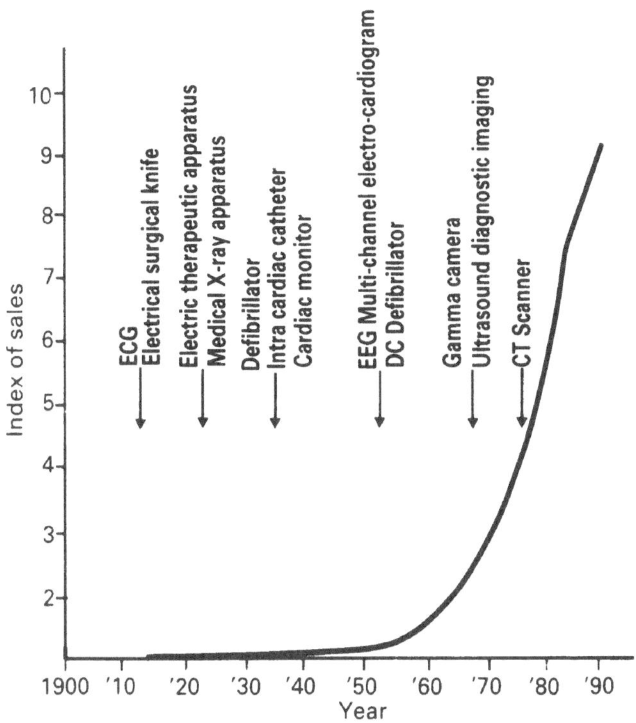

Source: Ministry of International Trade and Industry, *Denshi Kogyo Nenkan* (*Electronic Industry Yearbook*), 1987, p. 490

played a significant role in the progress of the medical industry. Knowledge that the peritoneum is semi-permeable dates back to the 1800s; efforts to apply this knowledge to the development of what is called peritoneal dialysis and to the manufacture of artificial kidneys dates from the early 1900s. Both approaches were improved during the 1940s and 1950s and the use of artificial kidneys and peritoneal dialysis have become commonplace in the treatment of chronic renal insufficiency. By the middle of the 1960s dialysis was thoroughly accepted in Japan and remains the preferred mode of treatment in a country which still has doubts about the ethics of organ transplantation. In 1967 dialysis was included in the health insurance fee schedule but patients were required at that time to make a fairly high co-payment for the treatment and it was burdensome for many chronic kidney patients. In 1971 a group of patients joined together to form a national association which campaigned for more financial assistance for their treatment. Government bowed to public pressure and since 1972 has picked up the co-payment.

Table 7.3 International comparison of dialysis patients, December 1975

Country	*Patients per million population*
Japan	126.2
Israel	103.1
USA	95.2
France	88.0
Switzerland	87.7
Luxembourg	81.9
Fed. Republic of Germany	81.8
Italy	75.1
Belgium	74.7
Canada	73.4
Netherlands	66.1
Denmark	57.8
Europe	45.5

Source: Kenji Maeda *et al.* 'The present situation and problems of the artificial kidney', *Ikakikaigaku Zasshi* (*Journal of Medical Machines and Apparatus*), 47, 7: 356, 1977

The numbers of chronic patients on dialysis and the number of artificial kidney machines have increased dramatically. There were 215 registered patients and 105 machines in 1968; 73,537 patients and 30,846 machines in 1986. This particular piece of treatment was and remains attractive to service-providers and equipment-makers alike; it is likely that there is an over-supply of kidney machines in the country. The health insurance schedule provides a generous reimbursement for a service that is now relatively straightforward and cheap to deliver. As we can see from Table 7.3 Japan recorded the highest ratio of chronic dialysis patients per 1 million population in the mid-1970s. Another life-saving device, the electric cardiac pacemaker has been less significant in Japan because cardiovascular diseases have not been so prevalent as in western nations. It is therefore worth noting that Japanese manufacturers have not made any substantial commitment to developing this kind of equipment and the Japanese medical establishment relies for the most part on imported models.

The development of the new generation of medical equipment since the late 1960s has required major investments by those companies willing to enter the field. They were rewarded by massive annual increases in sales through the 1970s, as we can see illustrated by Table 7.4.

However, the 1980s have seen production and sales figures slowing down partly because of saturation of the market (particularly for

Table 7.4 Trend in production of medical equipment, 1965–86

Year	*Amount (million yen)*	*Ratio over preceding year*
1965	8,503	
1966	7,604	89.4
1967	9,875	129.9
1968	12,114	122.7
1969	13,151	108.6
1970	19,247	146.6
1971	21,630	112.2
1972	23,591	109.1
1973	30,660	130.0
1974	35,823	97.4
1976	63,492	105.6
1977	88,379	139.2
1978	125,674	142.2
1979	164,665	131.0
1980	199,363	121.1
1981	212,901	106.8
1982	255,200	119.8
1983	293,049	114.8
1984	321,462	109.7
1985	340,772	106.0
1986	388,331	114.0

Source: Ministry of International Trade and Industry, *Denshi Kogyo Nenkan* (*Electronic Industry Yearbook*), Tokyo, 1987
Note: Reports from 41 firms until 1981, 74 firms in 1982, and 74 firms from 1983.

CT scanners for example) and partly because government policies to control health care costs are beginning to bite. The larger medical facilities are on the whole in a much better position to invest in new equipment and to provide the necessary operational costs (additional facilities, trained staff, budgets) than are the smaller clinics. It is among the latter in particular that sales are drying up. Having successfully tackled the question of drug costs within national medical expenditure the government next targeted fees for clinical diagnostic tests and especially tests which rely on complex electronic technology. Figure 7.2 illustrates projections for medical equipment expenditure as part of total national medical expenditure through to the end of the century.

An essential element in the government's goal of reducing its share of NME is encouragement of the entry of private enterprise in the health care field: a number of 'new' health care industries have emerged and some existing ones expanded since the mid-1980s. Not all of the new health industries are by any means based on high technology: many are often simply old-established industries with an added

Figure 7.2 Forecast for medical equipment production to the year 2000

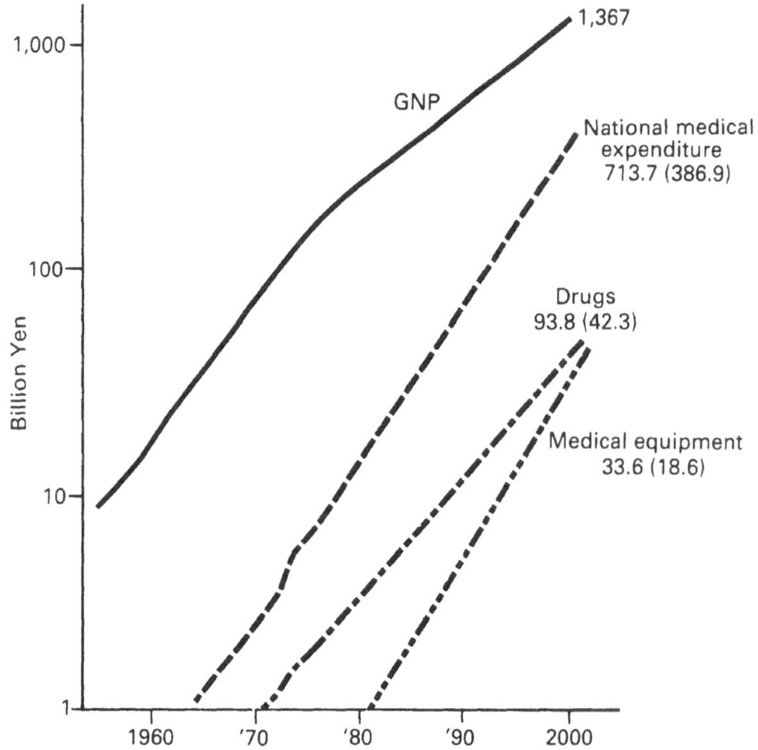

Source: Study Group on the Long-term Vision of Health and Welfare Problems, 'Conditions of establishment of new medical industry', *Tsusan Journal* (*Journal of International Trade and Industry*), April 1979
Notes: Figures in billion yen.
Figures in brackets are minimum predictions.

component designed to meet changing market needs or to meet gaps in existing service arrangements.

It has been estimated that in 1985 medical business had a value of 473,503 million yen of which 42.1 per cent was taken by the construction and engineering industries, and 32.5 per cent by private health insurance. Total revenue for 1988 was estimated at 773,800 million yen and will exceed 1 billion yen by 1990.

Hospital management

As hospitals of all shapes and sizes come to grips with the reality of the government's restraint on health financing they are being compelled to examine their management structures and practices with a view to obtaining improvements in efficiency. The provision of training programmes and consulting services is a fledgling but is a growing industry with an estimated 250 companies now in the market. Revenues have been estimated at 400 million yen in 1981, 500 million yen in 1982, 1,000 million yen in 1983, 15,000 million yen in 1984 and 30,000 million yen in 1985, with latent demand thought to be around 200,000 million yen.

Multi-hospital systems or chain hospitals

Hospital chains such as those found in the USA (e.g. Hospital Corporation of America, American Medicorp, Humana Inc., American Medical International, etc.) have not developed on a grand scale in Japan. This is mostly because the Medical Service Law requires that hospital boards are headed by a physician and that the hospital administrator is a physician; nor are hospitals allowed to be stock companies. Equally important the Japan Medical Association, which represents the interests of physician-owners of clinics and hospitals, has on the whole traditionally opposed the concept. A few groups do exist: the Tokushu-kai, for example, organized by a surgeon, Dr Torao Tokuda, is exceptionally well known for its efficient approach to the development and management of hospitals coupled with high-quality in-patient care and twenty-four-hour out-patient services – a rarity in Japan. The Tokushu-kai operates eleven hospitals throughout the country. Two of the large conglomerates (Sogoshosha), Mitsui Bussan and Itoh-Chu, have entered the area through joint ventures with American companies, the former with MPA Inc. and the latter with National Medical Enterprises. Daiei and Olympic Shopping Centre, both large nation-wide retailers, have become involved in hospital management. Although interest in this approach to hospital management is growing, growth has been slow with thirty hospitals so organized in 1983 and sixty in 1985.

Hospital staffing

A number of specialized employment agencies for temporary medical staff have been in operation since the start of the 1980s. Revenue has grown from 1,350 million yen in 1981 to 3,165 million yen in 1985. As many facilities seek to improve their efficiency they are looking to personnel costs: one method of cutting back is to reduce full-time nursing staff and utilize agency personnel as needed.

Hospital construction

Three huge construction companies have control of almost the whole hospital building industry which in 1985 was worth an estimated 199,000 million yen (up from 180,000 million yen in 1981). Taisei Construction had 52 per cent of the market share, Shimizu Construction 30 per cent and Takenaka Construction Company 14 per cent in 1984. In recent years these companies have expanded their range of services and in addition to the basic building construction they now offer comprehensive facilities planning and development services, including market research, site location, services planning, supply and logistics, operations and systems, simulation programmes for financial management, maintenance and other post-commissioning programmes. A new areá of interest for these companies is the potentially massive and highly lucrative market for facilities for elderly people, nursing homes, sheltered accommodation, and other types of long-term care facility, either as totally new developments or redevelopments of existing medical care facilities.

Hospital supplies and services

In the interests of efficiency and improved management many hospitals are contracting out a range of services: waste disposal, transportation, furniture and supplies, maintenance and catering services, including preparation of special diets. Smaller facilities often join together with other similar units nearby in order to obtain the most favourable rates for such services. Growth in this area has been good in the 1980s and total revenue in 1984 was estimated at 32,900 million yen. About 70 per cent of all medical facilities also refer their clinical tests to some eighty private laboratories, which operate around the country. As the government is exercising stricter monitoring of all diagnostic tests and the hospitals become more conscientious about the need for costly clinical tests, many of the labs are facing some reduction in annual revenues and they too are having to look into their own management practices.

Medical information systems

This comprises two components: hospital information systems and regional or area medical information systems. A total hospital information system includes medical care or patient information and hospital administration data. In Japan the greatest use of computer processing to date has been in the administration of salaries and wages and for patient billings. The use of computerized systems for patient records or for peer or utilization review is relatively undeveloped and offers great potential growth. Some 120 firms, mainly electric and electronic or computer companies, have entered and are expanding their hospital information systems business. NEC, Fuji Electric Company, Sanyo Electric, and Hitachi have cornered a 90 per cent share of the 45,000 million yen market in 1984. Regional or area medical information systems are mostly used by the public sector and computerization has been implemented on a fairly wide scale. The business was worth 500 million yen in 1982, 1,500 million yen in 1984, and 3,750 million yen in 1985.

Life care services

A relative newcomer to the health care industries, these encompass a broad range of health and health-related services such as routine or executive check-ups, telephone health counselling, private membership hospitals, and sheltered accommodation for senior citizens. Eight companies specialize in health check-ups, revenue from which was estimated at 1,250 million yen in 1985. The market is expanding, partly because preventive health care measures such as these are not included in normal health insurance, and popular concern about health is growing. Five firms offer telephone health information and counselling services. Takeda Medical Company, an affiliate of one of the largest pharmaceutical companies, Takeda, which has 30 per cent of total sales of digital haemodynamometers in the country, started a telephone information service on geriatric diseases as a joint venture with Kyorin University School of Medicine in July 1984 and recorded approximately 10,000 telephone enquiries in the first year of service.

Chugin Mansion Company accounts for more than 80 per cent of the market share in special apartments for elderly people. Several other firms are showing interest in this market, which had an estimated revenue of 4,000 million yen in 1984. Demand for such specialized accommodation is expected to grow as the proportion of elderly people in the population increases and because there is a huge shortage of nursing homes in Japan.

Equipment and services for domiciliary care

As part of its cost-containment policies, the government is emphasizing the expansion of home and community care services. Three types of self-care or treatment are included as health insurance benefits: insulin injection for diabetics (from 1981), injection of coagulant for haemophiliac patients (from 1983), and CAPD (Continuous Ambulatory

Peritoneal Dialysis) for renal insufficiency patients (from 1984). There are some 4,000 haemophiliac patients; 75 per cent of the total revenue of 3,000 million yen was shared by three pharmaceutical companies. Patients using CAPD numbered 800 and one pharmaceutical company monopolized the service for a revenue of 1,800 million yen.

Another category is equipment for bedridden patients such as adjustable beds, anti-bedsore mattresses, napkins, etc. Total revenue in this market in 1984 was 3,750 yen and 4,300 yen in 1985. Major suppliers are small or medium-sized specialist companies but more large firms are projected to enter this business, which will grow with the expected large increase in numbers of bedridden elderly patients.

Emergency medical services

Local public health departments and municipal fire departments are responsible for organizing emergency medical transportation services. Private firms do provide long-distance or international care and transfer services and one emergency medical care helicopter service has operated domestically since 1984. International Talisman Systems is preparing to start up international services based in Japan; two companies, Japan Medic Alert and SECOM, take care of the small-scale activity related to detection of accidents or emergency cases and provision of patient information and medical histories.

Private health insurance

People wishing to take out additional medical insurance cover have traditionally been able to do so by paying premiums for additional clauses in their regular life insurance policies. The American Family Company was the first to offer separate health insurance policies with its cancer insurance in 1974. At present there are four kinds of commercial health insurance coverage for (1) all types of disease; (2) coverage mainly for cancer; (3) coverage for cancer only, and (4) coverage for dementia. Ten companies have entered this independent health insurance market and total sales of policies were 72,300 million yen in 1981, 106,800 million yen in 1983, 128,200 million yen in 1984, and 153,800 million yen in 1985. It is thought that some 60 per cent of all households now carry some kind of commercial health insurance over and above their employment-related and mandatory insurance cover. As patient co-payment increases in line with government policy, a growth in demand for such additional cover is foreseen.

That the government clearly attaches some considerable importance to the growth of the business and industrial sectors of health and medical care can be seen by the establishment of a new section on Medical and Health Related Industry in the Ministry of Health and Welfare in early 1986. This section is charged with (1) conducting research into health-related industries, (2) exchanging information and liaising with other ministries which might be concerned with health-related industries, and (3) acting as an information centre working with medical institutions and those companies in health technology and industry.

References

1 *Health and Welfare Statistics in Japan, 1985*, Tokyo, Health and Welfare Statistics Association, 1987, pp. 112–13.
2 S. McKnight, *Japan's Pharmaceutical Industry No Longer Soaring*, Japan Economic Institute Report 45a, 22 November 1985, edited version in *American Chamber of Commerce Journal*, May 1986, pp. 75–84.
3 *Situation and Trends of Medical Insurance and Medical Supply in Japan, 1985*, Tokyo, National Federation of Health Insurance Societies, 1985, p. 105.
4 M. Reich, *SMON Disease*, Kodansha Encyclopaedia of Japan, 1984, p. 206.

Chapter eight

The health professions

The rapid growth in knowledge which has led to the development and application of new technology has contributed to immense improvements in medical care and opened up exciting new possibilities in the care and treatment of the sick. None the less the health care industry remains a labour-intensive one; it may be feasible to attach the sick individual to a machine for diagnosis, evaluation of progress, and treatment, but it is still necessary to ensure that trained and qualified people are involved in running the machines. Hence doctors make the decisions to initiate a course of therapy, nursing staff take charge of the daily care and comfort of the patient, and specialized technicians maintain and operate the plant and machinery. Of all the resource inputs in any health care system, staffing resources usually account for the lion's share of expenditure and this is valid no matter how the system is organized. In the United Kingdom some three-quarters of total health expenditure goes on salaries and wages; in the USA 30 per cent of total health expenditure covered physicians', dentists', and other professionals' services in 1982.[1] In Japan in the same year it has been estimated that remuneration of physicians in all types of facilities accounted for 48.8 per cent of expenditure.[2]

In this chapter therefore we shall be concerned with the people who deliver health care in Japan today: the professional organization, education and training, and working patterns within the health care delivery system of doctors, nurses, and other allied health workers. We hope too to shed some light on the nature of the role and status of each professional group within the community. While Japanese medical professionals bear many similarities to their counterparts elsewhere they undoubtedly also present characteristics which are distinctly Japanese.

The health care delivery system in Japan, more so than elsewhere, is one in which the medical profession remains the dominant one. Doctors, with their polite and reverential title of 'sensei' (teacher), play the central and key role in the provision of health care and are supported by other professionals, the nurses, therapists, technicians, and so forth whose status is definitely subordinate. In many countries social changes have had an impact on the health care delivery system and the role and status of the medical profession within it; the system is geared to the provision of effective, appropriate forms of treatment available and the doctor is now an important member of a health care team but is not necessarily always its leader. It is often thought that in Japan the patient is at the periphery of a professional and mysterious circle, the central point of which is the doctor. The Japanese on the whole prefer clearly delineated hierarchical relationships in which the duties and responsibilities of each participant are well known. When all the members of the group are fully conscious of their role and required contribution, there is no fretting or pulling against the ranking order; a team thus established will work well together to achieve common, mutually accepted goals. The medical team is headed by the doctor and works successfully because it is founded on these concepts; patients remain outside the privileged circle of professionals and must accept that it is working on their behalf and they will be the beneficiaries of the system.

The relationship between individual patient and doctor has likewise been distinguished to date by an unquestioning acceptance of the hierarchical ranking of the participants; this cultural preference and practice has certainly helped preserve the supremacy of the medical profession for so long. It is still, however, the physician who is a critical element in the utilization of available health care resources. We shall therefore look first at the medical profession in Japan, which currently comprises some 17 per cent of the total health care work-force in the country.

In 1984 there were an estimated 181,101 medical practitioners and 63,145 dentists in Japan.[3] The total number of doctors had grown by 41.8 per cent since 1970 and the physician:population ratio for the whole country has risen to 150.6 per 100,000 population (a 23 per cent increase) during the same time. Not unexpectedly the ratio is not uniform throughout the country: in the eleven major cities in 1982 for example, the ratio of doctors was 213.7 per 100,000 population, 141.5 in other cities, and 80.4 in small towns and villages. These figures offer confirmation of the continued concentration of doctors in the urban centres and have prompted renewed official concern about the urgency of rectifying the imbalance in the distribution of medical practitioners. While the Tokyo Metropolitan area enjoys the largest ratio of doctors for an individual city, 201.6 per 100,000, the prefectures immediately adjacent to the north and east have the smallest number of doctors per 100,000. Saitama and

Chiba Prefecture, with 86.4 and 93.6 per 100,000 population respectively, are the newest and most rapidly growing urban commuter centres for which adequate infrastructure, including medical services, has yet to be organized.

The uneven distribution of doctors is just one of the problems associated with the fee-for-service payment of doctors such as exists in Japan and there are as yet no mechanisms in the reimbursement system to correct this imbalance or induce doctors to move to under-doctored areas. The ratio for the country as a whole is not as generous as those in other developed countries but is deemed sufficient by the Ministry of Health and Welfare; official figures suggest too that if the present annual rate of increase in physician numbers is allowed to continue there will be 282,000 doctors by the year 2000, that is 200 per 100,000 population, a figure which is assessed as too high. Moreover if the present rural/urban maldistribution of doctors is not corrected, discrepancies in services provisions will be even more exaggerated than they are at present and will furthermore be out of step with expected requirements for medical services and care which will arise out of changes in population structure. Much of the growth in the medical work-force is in fact the result of deliberate government policy in the late 1960s, when a shortage of doctors encouraged the government to provide financial assistance to set up more medical schools, so that there would be at least one medical school in every prefecture. There was consequently a burgeoning in the number of medical schools and especially of the private schools and colleges, during the 1970s. By the end of 1981, 80 medical schools were enrolling close to 8,500 new students each year. Having arrived at acceptable numbers of doctors, government policy now is to limit the supply and it has established specialist committees to carry out detailed studies of future medical manpower requirements. In interim reports released to date, the Committee on Future Doctor Supply has recommended that annual growth in the number of doctors be pegged at 10 per cent until 1995 at least; that medical manpower supply be continuously reviewed; that measures be introduced to strengthen the medical work-force in public health services, and that the present nature of medical practice be modified so that it can better meet future needs.[4] The Committee has also voiced concern about the nature and quality of undergraduate medical training offered in the private medical schools in particular and has stressed the need to upgrade existing postgraduate and continuing education programmes.

The number of working women has shown a 2.8-fold increase in the past two-and-a-half decades and women now account for 35.6 per cent of the work-force.[5] However the proportion of women in senior or managerial positions, or in the professions, remains strikingly low; Japan trails a long way behind her fellow developed nations. Only in nursing, teaching, and pharmacy do women exceed 20 per cent of the total of employees; 3.1 per cent of lawyers and judges, 6.1 per cent of scientific researchers, and 10.9 per cent of doctors and dentists are women. In 1983 10.2 per cent of doctors were female and they are clustered, as is usually the case, in the 'female' specialties of obstetrics, gynaecology, and paediatrics; their numbers are high too in such specialties as ophthalmology, otolaryngology, and dermatology, which allow more organized scheduling of clinic sessions and on the whole involve fewer emergency procedures. Research studies have also shown that more women doctors then men doctors take up posts in public health services; again hours are regulated and conform to a conventional working day, hence allowing some time for the woman doctor to meet her other domestic and family commitments.

Medical practice

Japan has a long tradition of medical care in which ambulatory practice has played a dominant and vital role. Despite the trend towards greater reliance on hospital services, private medical practitioners remain the main provider of medical care and a key component in the health care system; their power and authority are reflected in the high social standing which the medical profession enjoys and takes advantage of still today. Even though doctors' incomes nowadays are not always guaranteed to reach the astronomical figures that were once the norm, the majority of doctors, particularly those who run their own practice or clinic, can look forward to a very comfortable income indeed. It says something about the profession that the Inland Revenue Service's league table of tax avoiders places the owners of private hospitals second only to Pachinko Parlour operators in volume of undeclared and taxable income.[6] The private practitioner in Japan is an entrepreneurial businessman who can usually find some lucrative loopholes, despite government limitations and regulations in the point-fee reimbursement scheme.

A medical graduate can expect to find employment in one of five major groups of practitioners. First, and by far the largest group, are the private practitioners where solo practice is the norm; there is a wide range in the nature and quality of services provided and in qualifications and levels of competence. Solo practice is precisely that: most doctors do not have secretarial help and hence cannot offer appointments; patients simply go to the clinic (or surgery) and wait their turn. Clinic hours are generally very long and a seven-hour day, six days a week is common for such single-handed doctors. In the absence of secretarial help spare time is devoted to practice administration and paperwork, including the preparation and processing of insurance claim forms. There are no legal obligations on such practitioners to provide emergency or after-hours cover to their patients and the majority do not do so. The majority of private doctors who work alone in this fashion are not quite general practitioners nor are they fully trained or certified specialists.

Medical practice varies according to locality – in rural areas and smaller towns and villages private practitioners offer something close to family physician or general practitioner services. In the cities, where there are more doctors, a private practitioner is more likely to offer a degree of specialist care. Most undergraduates elect to take some specialty training in the final year of their training; doctors setting up new practices advertise their expertise accordingly. Once established it is up to individual doctors to continue their specialist interests and to undertake any further training or refresher training. To do so may present some practical difficulties for those in solo practice, as attendance at conferences or training courses obviously takes them out of the practice, thus cutting into income. Given the number of hours worked and the isolation from professional colleagues which such practice necessarily entails, it is not surprising that many 'specialists' are either out of date or not true specialists at all. Private practices are well equipped with the most modern and elaborate diagnostic equipment available: it helps to attract new patients and conveys the appropriate aura of professional standing and competence. Private practitioners do not normally enjoy practice rights in hospitals and this has traditionally been one reason why they have pursued some specialty interest; by being in a position to offer specialist-level treatment, doctors have been able to keep their patients longer and therefore also to ensure income over a longer period of time. Once referred to a hospital for treatment both patient and income may well be lost.

A final and notable feature of private practice in Japan dates from the time when Chinese medicine was the only form of medical care: it is that doctors not only prescribe but also sell drugs to their patients. This practice causes raised eyebrows among foreign observers and within Japan herself in recent times has been the focus of heated debate and political action. The doctors have fought strongly, and so far successfully, to retain this right and not only on medical grounds. Recent government policies to rationalize the Drug Tariff Standards used in the point-fee-system have reduced the potential profit margin on each prescription, much to the disgruntlement of both the pharmaceutical industry and the medical profession; but drug-related activities – the prescription and sale of medication and giving injections – continue to contribute a substantial portion of any doctor's income. At present there are few mechanisms to monitor or control the level of drug dispensing by individual practitioners and disciplinary action is relatively unheard of. The significance of this practice can be seen in the data on drug costs as a part of total national medical care expenditure – 38.2 per cent in 1980 was the average figure but in general clinics drugs accounted for 44.2 per cent of total costs.[7] For any individual patient the cost of medication and injections can account for an average 50 per cent of the bill.

A second group of practitioners can be identified although they can be considered a logical extension of those working in solo practice: these are private doctors who have expanded their services and facilities to become clinics offering in-patient services and more specialized diagnostic and treatment services. Facilities with fewer than twenty beds are classified as clinics and there are some restrictions on the duration of patient stay. Such facilities once comprised the major part of the medical facilities in the country but their numbers are dwindling and the nature of services offered is changing.

A third group of doctors either own or are employed in the private hospitals which make up 80 per cent of all medical facilities in the country. The larger hospitals employ a full-time salaried medical staff which is grouped by specialty and divided by rank according to age and experience. The work of the staff is supervised by the medical superintendent or the medical director; often the latter is also the owner of the hospital which is then run as a family business. Japan has no true equivalent to the consultant post, so prestige and a higher income arrive with the gradual and orderly progression up the ladder to posts further up the hierarchy, head of a clinical unit, department chief, and perhaps eventually medical superintendent or director. The last position may not be a viable option in larger, prestigious hospitals, such as university affiliates, as the position may in effect be reserved for retired academic staff of the university: nor in the smaller hospitals where the owner is still an active member of the staff.

Like the private practices the hospitals exhibit a diverse range of facilities and quality of staff and services. If we can equate medical practice with Japanese business or industry, clearly many of the better facilities are comparable to the top one-third of Japanese companies. In such facilities the staff enjoy good social and sports amenities and excellent working conditions; the most recent diagnostic and treatment facilities are available; opportunities for study and research and further education are offered to ensure that

Table 8.1 Employment of physicians by service and sex, 1984

	Male		*Female*	
	N	*%*	*N*	*%*
Employers in hospitals	3,464	2.1	75	0.4
Employees in hospitals	56,637	34.9	5,564	29.5
Employers in clinics	58,795	36.2	6,091	32.3
Employees in clinics	6,872	4.2	2,748	14.6
Employees in medical school hospitals	30,008	18.5	3,198	17.0
Total in medical facilities	155,776	96.0	17,676	93.8
Employed in research institutions	3,548	2.2	195	1.0
Employed in administration	1,634	1.0	529	2.8
Others	360	0.2	43	0.2
Inactive (jobless or retired)	929	0.6	411	2.2
Total	162,247		18,854	

Source: Annual Survey of Physicians, Dentists and Pharmacists, Ministry of Health and Welfare, Tokyo, 1985

optimum skills prevail among the medical staff. Such hospitals tend to attract the better-qualified young doctors, who are encouraged to remain with the organization for the long term.

A fourth group of doctors works in the public sector in national and local government hospitals. These doctors are mostly specialists and hold full-time salaried positions. What they lose in income, by comparison with their colleagues in private practice, they gain in prestige and standing within both the medical community and the public at large. As Table 8.1 shows, the four groups described account for the majority of doctors in employment. A very small proportion of medical practitioners work full-time in public health services either as administrators or in clinical practice. Most doctors who work in public health centres are private practitioners who have a contract to work part-time, on average four or five days per month. A shortage of physicians who are engaged on a full-time and permanent basis in public health is a priority issue for health policy-makers, although measures introduced so far to encourage more doctors to enter this field of practice have met with very little success. Finally, a small number of doctors are primarily employed in teaching, research, and administration in universities, research institutes, and other public bodies.

In the annual survey of physicians, dentists, and pharmacists carried out by the Ministry of Health and Welfare, practising physicians are allowed to give multiple responses to questions about specialty practice and affiliation so it is not possible to state accurately the proportion of doctors engaged in general practice or working as obstetricians/gynaecologists and so forth. The majority (44.6 per cent) do claim that they primarily practise general medicine, 20 per cent practise paediatrics, 17 per cent general surgery, and 11.3 per cent gastro-enterology. In only seven specialties do women account for more than 10 per cent of the total number of active doctors: these were paediatrics, psychiatry, obstetrics, ophthalmology, ENT, dermatology, and anaesthesiology (further details are shown in Table 8.2).

However, this pattern of service is changing for reasons associated with the economics of health care delivery as well as the appropriateness of this medical model when patterns of disease and needs for services are changing. Keeping up with developments in medical science and practice and maintaining a current and effective knowledge of the newest developments in technology is an unrealistic proposition for single-handed practitioners: one which moreover may impose financial burdens which their practices cannot sustain unless they dilute their standards of care and service. The cost of investing in the latest diagnostic and therapeutic equipment to support the goal of a 'specialist' practice cannot be recouped. Similar difficulties face the owners and staff of clinics and small hospitals. Given the nature of the most common diseases today many medical practitioners are waking up to the fact that their effectiveness is ultimately limited and that the new technology and 'specialist' treatment may well be irrelevant to the needs of the bulk of their clientele. Medical practice is therefore changing in Japan just as it is elsewhere. Among younger practitioners general practice as a family physician is increasingly considered a more viable and sensible approach; government policy to modify the point-fee system is reinforcing this by providing reimbursement for items of service which were previously excluded, as they were preventive health measures rather than concrete items of medical care. Similarly, restricting the reimbursement for high-technology diagnostic and therapeutic services to certain approved procedures or facilities is also forcing some reassessment on the part of the medical profession about what constitutes proper and relevant medical practice. The principal motivating factor behind the government's moves has been the control of total health care spending, and particularly the public sector part of it; the net effect has been some element of rationing of high-technology services and as a spin-off it is introducing some much-needed changes in attitudes and practice on the part of the medical profession. With perhaps fewer facilities offering highly specialized up-to-the-minute technological medicine, and the clinics and smaller hospitals offering general medical care more attuned to community needs, the once fuzzy situation and lack of distinction between specialist and general medical practice will be clarified.

Table 8.2 Number of physicians by sex and specialty, 1984

Specialty	*Number of physicians*			*% by specialty*			*% by sex*	
	Male	*Female*	*Total*	*Male*	*Female*	*Total*	*Male*	*Female*
General medicine	69,995	7,345	77,340	44.9	41.6	44.6	90.5	9.5
Respiratory medicine	8,251	538	8,789	5.3	3.0	5.1	93.9	6.1
Gastro-enterology	18,840	748	19,588	12.1	4.2	11.3	96.2	3.8
Cardiovascular medicine	11,576	662	12,238	7.4	3.7	7.1	94.6	5.4
Paediatrics	29,716	5,310	35,026	19.1	30.0	20.2	84.8	15.2
Psychiatry	6,498	821	7,319	4.2	4.6	4.2	88.8	11.2
Neurology	5,365	585	5,950	3.4	3.3	3.4	90.2	9.8
Neuro-medicine	2,291	199	2,490	1.5	1.1	1.4	92.0	8.0
General surgery	30,259	429	30,688	19.4	2.4	17.7	98.6	1.4
Orthopaedic surgery	16,126	268	16,394	10.4	1.5	9.5	98.4	1.6
Plastic surgery	886	77	963	0.6	0.4	0.6	92.0	8.0
Cosmetic surgery	150	11	161	0.1	0.1	0.1	93.2	6.8
Neurosurgery	3,944	47	3,991	2.5	2.3	2.3	98.8	1.2
Respiratory surgery	845	6	851	0.5	0.0	0.5	99.3	0.7
Cardio-thoracic surgery	1,339	13	1,352	0.9	0.1	0.8	99.0	1.0
Paediatric surgery	1,037	95	1,132	0.7	0.5	0.7	91.6	8.4
Obstetrics/gynaecology	10,998	1,193	12,181	7.1	6.7	7.0	90.2	9.8
Gynaecology	1,110	118	1,228	0.7	0.7	0.7	90.4	9.6
Obstetrics	1,991	316	2,307	1.3	1.8	1.3	86.3	13.7
Ophthalmology	5,267	2,773	8,040	3.4	15.7	4.6	65.6	34.5

Table 8.2 contd.

Specialty	*Number of physicians*			*% by specialty*			*% by sex*	
	Male	*Female*	*Total*	*Male*	*Female*	*Total*	*Male*	*Female*
ENT	6,650	1,221	7,871	4.3	6.9	4.5	84.5	15.5
Broncho-oesophogy	1,469	88	1,557	0.9	0.5	0.9	94.3	5.7
Dermatology	11,160	1,400	12,560	7.2	7.9	7.2	88.9	11.1
Urology	7,011	119	7,130	4.5	0.7	4.1	98.3	1.7
STD	1,525	41	1,566	1.0	0.2	0.9	97.4	2.6
Proctology	3,547	51	3,598	2.3	0.3	2.1	98.6	1.4
Physiotherapy	6,425	199	6,624	4.1	1.1	3.8	97.0	3.0
Radiology	11,238	537	11,775	7.2	3.0	6.8	95.4	4.6
Anaesthesiology	3,905	545	4,450	2.5	3.1	2.6	87.8	12.2
General	1,179	73	1,252	0.8	0.4	0.7	94.2	5.8
Others	1,387	95	1,482	0.9	0.5	0.9	93.6	6.4
Not known	86	9	95	0.1	0.1	0.1	90.4	9.6

Source: Report on Survey of Physicians, Dentists and Pharmacists, Statistics and Information Department, Ministry of Health and Welfare, Tokyo, 1985
Note: Total numbers for each specialty include multiple and dual responses

Medical education

As yet Japan's system of medical education is formally organized only as far as undergraduate medical training is concerned; postgraduate education is still very loosely structured.

There is a phenomenon in Japan known as the 'Kyoiku mama' (the education mama), who is a much satirized and caricatured figure, a favourite butt of television comedy shows. Her pre-eminence in the satire stakes is a sure indication that behind the fun and humour there lies a bitter and awesome reality. The ultimate goal of the education mama and the motivating force of her life is to achieve academic success for her children, success being defined as getting them into the best university in the country as this will guarantee future success and security in the shape of employment with one of the top corporations or one of the elite ministries of government. Tokyo University, known as Todai, sits atop the country's university pyramid. Founded in 1877 it was the first comprehensive university in the country and opened with four departments – law, medicine, liberal arts, and the natural sciences. It was designated an Imperial University in 1886 and until the 1890s its faculty members were mostly Europeans and Americans. Todai now has the prestige and aura of Oxbridge, Harvard, and Yale all rolled into one; it has produced most of Japan's prime ministers and continues to spawn the country's leading political figures, economists, bureaucrats, and leaders of commerce and industry. Kyoto, the second Imperial University, was established in 1897; during the latter years of the nineteenth century the government set up many institutions of higher education called 'Senmon Gakko' (professional schools) thus setting down the pattern for the multi-tiered structure of higher education still in force today. The state and public universities remain at the top of the educational hierarchy although there are not enough of them to take in all aspiring students. The gap between demand and places has long been filled by the private universities and colleges, which like their public counterparts have a hierarchy of quality. Keio (1890) and Waseda (1902) Universities in Tokyo head the private sector and below this first division is a vast and motley collection of institutions offering different types and quality of higher education and training.

Getting into the right university is a costly, fraught, and often destructive process which for many starts in the kindergarten years, when right-minded and ambitious parents ensure that their children enter the right kindergarten, which will lead to the right elementary school, and so on up to high school, and on into the best universities. For those who can afford private education the aim is get into

Keio or Waseda and they and other private universities operate affiliated kindergarten, elementary, and secondary schools which parallel the state system. With examinations at every stage in the process school years for the average Japanese child are not a time of exploration, discovery, and fun so much as a relentless grind of rote learning, assimilation of fact, and learning to conform.

Students aspiring to the medical profession must survive the same grim process in an exacerbated form as the academic requirements for the medical schools of the state universities are notoriously high and success in the medical school entrance examinations is the only method of selection for entry. For the majority of private medical schools entry is also based on academic qualifications and performance in entrance examinations. A number of private schools were the focus of scrutiny during the 1970s because of the high fees charged and too much flexibility regarding the necessary minimum entrance requirements: prospective students whose parents donated substantial gifts and funds to the institution often found it much easier to gain admittance than did applicants with better academic records but not so much money. Tuition fees at private medical schools remain much higher than at state schools and an entrance fee may also be required. Not surprisingly medicine remains a profession for the well-to-do in Japan; 30 per cent of medical school entrants are the children of medical practitioners and the practice of attending the same school as one's parent is strong. Annual intake to medical schools has averaged 8,000 students in recent years. The number and proportion of women entrants to medical schools has grown steadily; they accounted for 18 per cent of all entrants in 1983 but differences in male:female ratios between the public and private universities remained (see Table 8.3). In 1986 there were eighty-three medical schools throughout the country: forty-one national, nine municipal, and twenty-eight private institutions. A complete listing is given in Appendix 3. The first modern medical school, Tokyo University Medical School, had its origins in the Vaccination Centre set up in Edo in 1858, and was formally established as one of the first faculties of the University of Tokyo in 1877; the second school, at Kyoto, opened in 1897. Medical education in the 1870s and 1880s was very much a copy of the German medical education system of the day in keeping with government policy to introduce western medicine modelled on the German system. There was a three-year pre-medical period followed by five years of clinical training. In these early days another option for medical training was via an apprenticeship or vocational training programme in the government or approved hospitals. For some time doctors who were licensed to practise in this manner were in the

Table 8.3 Trend of entrants to medical schools by sex and category of school

Year		*National*		*Prefectural and Municipal*		*Private*		*Total*	
		N	*%*	*N*	*%*	*N*	*%*	*N*	*%*
1965	M	1,824	91	546	91	1,001	85	3,371	89
	F	188	9	57	9	175	15	420	11
	T	1,012		603		1,176		3,791	
1970	M	2,100	91	571	90	1,522	87	4,193	89
	F	207	9	63	10	223	13	493	11
	T	2,307		634		1,745		4,686	
1980	M	3,911	89	571	83	2,613	81	7,095	85
	F	499	11	115	17	631	19	1,245	15
	T	4,410		686		3,244		8,340	
1983	M	3,855	84	536	79	2,515	79	6,906	82
	F	730	16	143	21	686	21	1,559	18
	T	4,585		679		3,201		8,465	

Source: Medical Education, vol. 16, no. 2, Feb. 1985, Ministry of Education Statistics

majority, but their status was held to be inferior to that of the graduates of the universities and colleges, even though the latter were fewer in number.[8] With the Medical Practitioner Law of 1906, licensing of medical practitioners was restricted to graduates of universities or colleges which were subject to regulation by the education authorities.

Up until the end of the Second World War licence to practise as a doctor was automatically conferred on any graduate who had successfully passed the internal examinations set by the various universities and colleges. In addition to the seven Imperial universities, medical education was also provided in the professional schools, the Igaku Senmon Gakko, which had been set up in order to develop as rapidly as possible sufficient training facilities to produce enough physicians qualified in western medicine. This group of schools grew especially quickly during the Second World War to cope with a drastic shortage of doctors.

A school worthy of special mention was started in 1900 by Yoshioka Yayoi, a pioneer woman doctor who was concerned that opportunities for women to join the new profession were limited. Only after a twenty-year campaign was the Tokyo Women's Medical School (Tokyo Joigakko) officially recognized and given full accreditation, thus granting license to practise to its graduates on equal terms with the graduates of other institutions. The school was renamed the Tokyo Women's Medical College (Tokyo Joshi Ika Daigaku) after the war and continues as the only all-female medical college in the country. Entry is difficult as it enrols only fifty students each year; academic standards are high and there is no doubt that a prior connection with the college is a valuable asset for a potential student.

Medical education was also tackled in the education reforms carried out by the Occupation forces. The pre-war differences in medical education provided at the Imperial Universities and the professional schools were eliminated; a number of the latter facilities were closed down and some were upgraded to the level of the universities so that the type and quality of medical training became more uniform.

The basic undergraduate medical course has not been radically altered since that time although some amendments have been made in the examination and licensing procedures. Following twelve years of general education and after passing the necessary entrance examinations the Japanese medical student takes a sequentially organized programme consisting of two years' pre-medical course work in the natural sciences, humanities, and social sciences, followed by four years of para-clinical and clinical sciences.

Some schools now introduce subjects such as anatomy in the second pre-medical year. Students receive from one to two years of practical work with patients on the hospital wards during the course. In the past such clinical work was done only in special units of the out-patient clinic: students often graduated without having seen a hospital in-patient.

In order to be registered as legally qualified medical practitioners, the students must pass the national medical examination set by the Ministry of Health and Welfare. Until 1968 this examination could be taken only after students had obtained their medical degree and completed a one-year internship at a medical school teaching hospital or hospital designated by the ministry. Difficulties in organizing internships eventually led to the abolition of this system. The examination for licensing can now be taken by the medical graduate without any further compulsory education or training; once registered, new doctors are free to practise medicine in the setting of their choice. A two-year residency period in an approved hospital is recommended for medical graduates but it is not obligatory. However some 80 per cent of newly graduated physicians receive residency training, the majority electing to do so in their university teaching hospital.[9]

Strong allegiance to one's university is the norm and there is a well-developed and highly intricate system of patronage in medical schools by which the clinical professors arrange for the future deployment of departmental graduates. The medical schools maintain close links with the university teaching hospitals first and foremost, but they also have good connections with definite but not necessarily formal networks of 'affiliated' hospitals – affiliated in the sense that they are run and/or staffed by graduates of the same university. Hospital department heads will turn first to their Alma Mater and clinical professor for recommendations when looking for new staff.

Postgraduate education and training

Neither the government nor the medical profession itself is entirely satisfied with present arrangements for the postgraduate and continuing education of doctors, but efforts to reorganize it have to proceed slowly in order to accommodate the many groups and viewpoints concerned. Japan does not have any bodies which correspond to the specialty colleges or learned societies such as those found in the United Kingdom, Australia, or the USA and which historically have controlled entry into a specialty by determining the contents of training programmes, setting minimum standards of professional conduct, and conducting appropriate entrance and qualifying examinations. It is through such bodies that specialist groups within the medical profession have been able to ensure that minimum standards of skill apply. The specialist training provided in the past in Japan has been poorly organized and in the absence of nationally determined standards has produced diffuse levels of skill and competence.

There is a postgraduate training programme, the Igaku Hakase, introduced in 1957, which provides some structured programmes of advanced training within the medical schools. Lasting four to six years this can be equated with a Ph.D in medicine and it is usually pursued by students who plan to remain in university departments or to join the staff of teaching hospitals or specialized facilities. The precise nature of the course for each specialty varies from one school to the next. Course content is determined by the professorial body and commonly reflects the special research or other interests of the professor or other influential members of the faculty. Each medical school organizes its own curriculum and sets its own examinations; national guidelines apply for national examinations. Other medical graduates who join hospital residency programmes receive a two-year training programme rotating through all the clinical departments of the hospital, and thereafter they can elect to remain and work in the department of their choice, if an opening exists. Again each hospital organizes its own training curriculum and there are no national examinations which can measure student competence against any standards for the country as a whole. Hospital specialists are therefore more likely to have acquired their knowledge and expertise by dint of practice and practical learning from their seniors than through academic or theoretical training. Once licensed to practise doctors may enter general or specialist practice without any further obligatory formal training; nor are they required to attend further training or refresher courses during the course of their career. Those who do do so voluntarily and at their own expense.

The Japan Medical Association and its local affiliates (the town, city, and prefectural associations) constitute the leading health care professional group in the country. Local and prefectural associations enjoy considerable autonomy; a doctor must join a prefectural association in order to be eligible to become a member of the national body. In the past the JMA has functioned primarily as a political pressure group to represent and protect the interests of doctors within the community. Its activities in areas of professional standards and practice have been less significant. The Japan Medical Society is the association's scientific and technical arm although it has no real authority or regulatory powers. Other professional groups include the Society of Obstetricians and Gynaecologists, the Japan Paediatric Society, and so on.[10] Research and advisory groups centred on university departments take some responsibility for professional standards and play an important role in issuing guidelines of conduct and practice, especially in areas where there may be ethical or moral problems. The Liver Transplant Research Group headed by an Osaka University professor is an example of this kind of group. The professional associations have research and education committees and they advise accordingly but they have no regulatory or statutory responsibilities. The medical schools play a significantly more important role in this regard. On the whole it is a fair assessment to say that the medical profession in Japan is highly self-regulated and not open to public scrutiny. Despite occasional lapses high ethical standards have prevailed. There is a growing realization that a more structured approach is becoming necessary if the profession is to be properly constituted in terms of specialists and general practitioners for the future.

In a 1985 survey carried out by the Ministry of Health and Welfare doctors and nurses at one hundred government medical facilities reported that only 5.4 per cent of patients who had died of cancer in 1983 were aware that they had the disease; the majority of patients (54.3 per cent) did not know, and 20 per cent were 'uncertain' about what they were suffering from.[11] This high proportion of patients was apparently ignorant about the real nature of their illness because their doctors had not disclosed the facts to them. In yet another survey however, the ministry interviewed

28,000 men and women on the subject of stomach cancer, the leading form of the disease in the country.[12] Among the respondents, 45 per cent wanted to be told all the facts about the disease should they get it, 11.5 per cent said they would want their doctor to 'hint' at the truth, 20 per cent did not want to know the truth, and the remainder were undecided on the issue. There were differences in response by age: more men than women (60 per cent compared to 53 per cent) indicated that they preferred to know the whole truth. Most interesting was the finding that some two-thirds of all respondents believed the disease to be curable.

The concept of the patient's right to know is not widely understood, let alone accepted or practised in Japan. The stability of the doctor–patient relationship in the past has depended on a delicate balance of patient confidence in the medical profession and a finely tuned sense of the value of prevailing hierarchical order. Patients have accepted what the doctor did (or more usually did not) tell them, because the doctor definitely knew best.

The two surveys mentioned above not only highlight the disconcerting discrepancy in thinking and attitudes towards disease between the medical profession and the general public, but also confirm the conservatism which marks the medical profession as a whole in the country today. Probably the majority of doctors maintain a protective and paternalistic attitude towards their patients. In the past the doctor did not discuss the patients' problems with them either in much detail or in specific terms which the patients might understand. Vague intimations about the matter accorded with the Japanese ideal of tacit communication and if these were followed by some fairly brisk reassurance and suitable medication the patient could be sent away feeling confident: this in turn would help the healing process. Until recent times this approach suited all concerned. It preserved the mystique of the profession and as long as doctors were dealing with relatively 'straightforward' diseases which could be treated and cured it was not inappropriate. However the power of medicine has taken something of a battering; the effectiveness of the traditional approach has diminished in the face of chronic diseases which are not so susceptible to traditional clinical practice. 'Cures' are more difficult despite the application of the latest in technology and scientific intervention: patients have started to look for something else from their doctors. The new vulnerability of the medical profession applies not only to Japan of course, but in Japan tales of over-prescribing and unnecessary procedures, documented reports of malpractice, inefficiency, and corruption among institutions and individual practitioners alike, all have added to public unease and dealt a considerable blow to the inherent trust which for so long characterized the relationship between the medical profession and the general public. Growing public awareness and the availability of more information have heightened concerns about such matters as misdiagnosis and these are not assuaged when doctors simply resort to more and more diagnostic tests which cost a lot of money but do not in the end seem to result in any relief of the problem.

Nurses

Nurses make up approximately 60 per cent of the health work-force in Japan; they are grouped into four principal categories according to the nature and level of their education and training, specific skills and functions in the health care delivery system. Clinical nurses, the equivalent of registered nurses, are the largest group (47 per cent of the nursing work-force) while assistant nurses are almost as many in number.[13] Specialist midwives totalled just over 26,000 in 1982 and were 4.3 per cent of the work-force; with 19,137 members, the public health nurses were the smallest category. There is a small number of male nurses in the country, most of whom work in hospitals and particularly the mental hospitals. Male midwives are prohibited by law in Japan.

As with doctors the geographical distribution of nurses is not uniform throughout the country and the two prefectures with the lowest ratio of nurses per 100,000 population are also those with the lowest doctor:population ratios, namely Saitama and Chiba (close to Metropolitan Tokyo) which had 20.1 and 21.2 nurses per 100,000 population respectively in 1982. Tokyo, which had one of the highest doctor:population ratios, is not so well supplied with nurses and ranked in the bottom half of all prefectures with 35.8 nurses per 100,000 population.

There are some expected differences in the location of work among the four categories. The public health nurses are employed almost exclusively in local authority health programmes, working out of health centres and clinics where they provide child health care and check-ups, carry out preventive health care, and work in home nursing services. A few are employed in hospitals and private clinics or in industrial and occupational nursing.

Public health nurses are registered clinical nurses who have taken the one-year public health nurse training course and passed the national examinations. Close to half of all midwives now work in hospitals, almost twice the proportion who did so in 1970. One-third of practising midwives either own or work in maternity clinics; as a result of changes in the nature and pattern of maternal and child health (MCH) service delivery this group has shown a sharp decline in numbers – more than 50 per cent of all midwives worked in this setting in 1970. The remaining 16 per cent of midwives work in clinics, most of which are obstetrics/gynaecology clinics. The proportion who have worked in this setting has remained fairly constant at approximately 16 per cent in the last two decades. Midwifery is the oldest of the nursing professions in Japan. Indigenous midwives practised in the Edo era and the first training school for midwives was set up in 1876 in the Tokyo Prefectural Hospital, predating the first Nurses Training School by some eight years. The first regulations governing the licensing and employment of midwives were enacted in 1899.

Like their counterparts elsewhere in the world, midwives have seen the nature of their practice undergo quite dramatic changes, especially in the past thirty years when Japan too has seen the control and management of childbirth become the domain of the medical profession. The midwifery service probably enjoyed its greatest success and prestige in the 1960s, when government accelerated the public MCH programme through the expansion of MCH centres. Since the 1970s most midwives now function in the hospitals handling antenatal care, normal labour and delivery under the supervision of the medical staff. Like British midwives, Japanese midwives undergo the full three-year training to become a registered nurse followed by the one-year course in midwifery.

The basic nurse's education and training programme (in some respects) is similar to the English programme. Graduates of senior high school (18 years old) take a three-year full-time training course at a nursing school and must pass the national examination, which is set up by the Ministry of Health and Welfare, in order to obtain their licence to practice. Unlike the British system however, nurses are not paid employees of the hospital while they are in training and do not put in as much time on the wards. They are students in the proper meaning of the word and the training course is organized so that academic course work is interspersed with periods of practical work on the wards. When they do work on the wards student nurses are usually allocated one or two patients only, they do not do night duty, and they are throughout closely supervised by the senior nursing staff. Entry as an assistant nurse is via a different route: this grade of nursing is open to 16-year-old graduates of junior high school. Recent applicants include senior high school leavers, who take a two-year programme in schools of nursing or, more usually, junior colleges. It is the local government at the prefectural level which sets the qualifying examinations for this grade. Assistant nurses are licensed to provide nursing care under the direction of physicians, dentists, or (clinical) nurses. The grade can be assessed

Table 8.4 Category of nursing schools and student capacity, 1984

Ownership	*Number*	*Student capacity*
National (MHW)	139	15,850
National (others)	89	10,735
Local government		
Prefectural	337	36,455
Municipal	154	13,216
Red Cross	38	3,760
Other semi-public and private (JMA, etc)	888	99,007
Total	1,645	179,023

Source: Statistical Data on Nursing Service in Japan, 1984, compiled under supervision of Nursing Division, Health Policy Bureau MHW, Tokyo, 1985, p. 34

as corresponding to that of an enrolled nurse.

There were 1,645 nursing schools, offering just over 179,000 places in 1984. Some of the schools are affiliated with the universities or are a part of university medical schools: other specialized or independent schools of nursing are associated with the social insurance organizations, or hospital groups such as the Red Cross. Sponsorship of all the schools is shown in Table 8.4.

Of the clinical nurses, 80 per cent work in hospitals, less than 15 per cent in clinics, and the remainder are engaged in nurse education and training and research. The deployment of assistant nurses is slightly different: 65 per cent work in hospitals and 34 per cent in clinics. When we look more closely at the statistics on deployment of these two categories of nursing staff, and particularly at the number of nurses per 100 hospital beds, some illuminating differences emerge according to the category of the sponsoring body (i.e. whether the hospital is a public or private one). The statistics moreover seem to add some weight to impressionistic evidence and popular thinking that hospitals suffer from a shortage of nurses. The ratio of all nursing personnel, that is midwives, nurses, assistant nurses, and unqualified nurse aides was 37.7 per 100 beds in 1982. Omitting the nurse aides and dealing only with trained and qualified staff, the ratio dropped to 31.0 per 100 beds. However, depending on the category of ownership, there were were more or fewer qualified nurses and striking differences in the ratios: see Tables 8.5 and 8.6. Within the semi-public and private sector moreover the ratios vary considerably: the Red Cross hospitals have a total of 44.0 qualified nursing staff for 100 beds, the largest private institutions have between 30 and 40 qualified staff for 100 beds, the majority of privately owned hospitals (6,678 out of 9,387 and almost three-

Table 8.5 Ratio of nursing staff to hospital beds, 1982

Ownership category	*Ratio per 100 beds*
National (MHW)	29.9
National (others)	46.8
Local government	43.1
Semi-public	40.9
All private	26.3

Source: Statistical Data on Nursing Service in Japan, 1984, compiled under supervision of Nursing Division, Health Policy Bureau, MHW, Tokyo, 1985, pp. 20–1
Note: Nursing staff means midwives, nurses, and assistant nurses; nurse aides are omitted.

Table 8.6 Deployment of nursing staff, 1982

Ownership category	*Midwives and nurses (%)*	*Assistant nurses (%)*	*Nurse aides (%)*
National (MHW)	66.1	20.5	13.1
National (others)	83.5	8.9	7.6
Local government	65.0	28.5	6.6
Semi-public	62.1	26.1	11.8
All private	34.9	41.5	23.6

Source: Statistical Data of Nursing Service in Japan, 1984, compiled under supervision of Nursing Division, Health Policy Bureau MHW, Tokyo, 1985, pp. 20–1

quarters of the total) had just 22.9 qualified nursing staff per 100 beds.

Furthermore the private hospitals employ a higher proportion of assistant nurses and unqualified nurse aides than do the public facilities. Private hospitals commonly do not employ their nursing staff on a full-time basis moreover, and it is common practice to hire agency nurses as and when patient numbers require more staff. The services of these nurses are paid for out of the extra charge fees levied from patients. By keeping full-time or permanent staff to the absolute minimum hospital operators keep a lid on total running costs.

Among private facilities there is a range of figures; ratios for the institutionally owned hospitals are more generous than those for the small and individually owned ones. The latter make up 87 per cent of this sector and have a nursing staff made up of 26 per cent midwives and clinical nurses, 47.6 per cent assistant nurses, and 26.4 per cent nurse aides, so the highest qualified staff group is outnumbered by those with lower qualifications or no qualifications at all. Together the statistics cited above offer some substantiation for the concern within the profession and among the general public that too many hospitals are inadequately or improperly staffed, and that nurses are overworked and stretched beyond the level and capacity for which they have been trained.

Post-basic training courses and opportunities to acquire specialist training have not been widely developed in Japan; clinical nurses eventually opt to remain on medical and surgical wards after several years of rotating through all the departments of a hospital. The exact structure of hospital nursing administration is quite varied because of the varied nature of all Japanese hospitals. In the larger, usually public facilities such as the national hospitals or the large facilities affiliated with social insurance bodies or groups such as the Red Cross, nursing administration is more structured with a director of nursing taking charge of all aspects of nursing administration including staffing, services planning, and overseeing education and training functions. In most smaller organizations nursing staff may be under the supervision of the medical superintendent, with a sister in charge responsible at ward level. In these facilities nurses have no real input into management of services.

According to popular mythology nurses in Japan are hard-working and long-suffering; they must be servile and respectful to doctors and administrators; their financial rewards are meagre and not commensurate with the role they play in caring for the sick. Nurses' professional status and skills are unrecognized: they are the unsung heroines of the hospital world. Certainly the profession has suffered from low esteem and status; in a health care system which for over one hundred years has placed the doctor in a central and pivotal role with all other health care professionals viewed as mere acolytes, nurses have suffered twofold discrimination. The nurse's role has been viewed as an extension of the woman's role in Japan: the education and training of nurses has not substantially altered since 1947, a factor which has not helped the nurse's own goal of enhancing the status of the profession.

The two-level training and subsequent overlapping of functions and responsibilities on the wards have been unsatisfactory; the medical profession has been happy to exploit the situation as hospital owners have been able to employ more staff in the assistant nurse grade thus keeping up overall numbers and meeting minimum legal requirements while keeping costs down.

The profession is keen to eliminate the assistant nurse grade for the future and to introduce a uniform four-year basic training programme for all entrants to the profession. Upgrading the professional status of nurses and modernizing their education and training are key issues of policy for the Japanese Nursing Association (JNA), one of the more lively of the health care industry's professional groups in the country. The JNA believes too that nurses should have a greater say in medical and health care administration and in planning for future health care services. The nurses feel that they are in closer contact with patients and often in a better position to assess their needs. The nurses hold that the role of nursing staff will become more rather than less critical in the years to come and that a more cogent representation of their views is needed to ensure that Japan gets the right kind of health care provisions.

Other health professionals

In all an estimated 2 million professional men and women work in health care in Japan; about 1.5 million have national or prefectural licences to practise and are members of accredited professional organizations. In addition to the doctors, nurses, and dentists Japan's health professionals include pharmacists, clinical radiographers, laboratory technicians, physical and occupational therapists, dental hygienists and dental technologists and dietitians. These allied health professionals in Japan still play a much more secondary role to the physicians than is perhaps the case now in many other countries. This is partly the result of the historical development of these professions and a reflection of the continued dominance of the doctor in the Japanese health system. Early practitioners were trained essentially as assistants to the doctors; their training was not systematized or founded on any national guidelines and they received no formal qualifications. It is only in the last twenty or thirty years that formal training programmes, curricula, and state examinations for the varied allied health professionals have gradually been established, and the nature of their practice and responsibilities been defined.

Training for allied health professionals is normally provided in colleges of medical sciences which are attached to and normally on the same campus as a medical school. As with doctors a well-established old boys' network operates to ensure that the training institutes can place their graduates in the right hospitals. The college staff organize placement prior to final examinations and knowing the ability and skills of their students they can generally assure a good match between individual graduates and prospective employer needs. It is widely known that many colleges set their own quotas for getting graduates into the best medical facilities: this means that the students are careful in their choice of college. Hospitals tend to recruit particular types of allied health professionals from the same training school. The system ensures employment for graduates and on the whole suits all the participants but as with the medical profession it does tend to limit professional mobility and inhibit the

Table 8.7 Legislation of health professions

Medical Services Law	1948
Medical Practitioners Act	1948
Dental Practitioners Act	1948
Dental Hygienist Act	1948
Public Health Nurses, Midwives and Nurses Act	1948
Dental Technologists Act	1955
Pharmaceutical Affairs Act	1960
Pharmacists Act	1960
Physiotherapists and Occupational Therapists Act	1965
Orthoptists Act	1966
Clinical Radiographic Technologists and Clinical X-Ray Technicians Act	1968
Law relating to Massagists, Acupuncturists and Moxabuctionists	1970
Judo-manipulators Law	1970
Clinical Laboratory Technologists and Hygienic Laboratory Technicians Act	1970
Ortho-prothesists Act	1987
Clinical Engineers Act	1987

Source:

introduction of new blood into the hospitals.

Speech therapists, clinical psychologists, medical social workers, and health and hospital administrators are professional groups who are playing a greater role in the delivery of health care in Japan but as yet they have not received national recognition in the form of national training standards and qualifications. There are frustrations among all allied health professionals about their subordinate role to doctors: most of the legislation for their qualifications for example usually starts by describing the limitations of their activities under the supervision of physicians. Lip service is paid to the growing importance of the team work approach in health care but the proper organizational structures and the development of democratic and efficient health care teams by the different health professionals, together with co-ordination between health and social welfare professionals remain thorny topics in health care administration in Japan today, (see Table 8.7).

There are approximately 120,000 practitioners of traditional therapies at work in Japan and they include acupuncturists, moxacauterists, finger-pressure therapists (shiatsu-shi), judo-orthopaedists (judo-seifukushi), and chiropractors. Like the practitioners of 'western' medicine, their education and training is now covered by well-established curricula and training programmes and they must pass prefectural examinations to obtain a licence to practise. They are not allowed to do surgery nor to prescribe certain kinds of medication. For the most part treatment by traditional therapists is not included in the various health insurance schemes and patients must pay for their services out of their own pockets. Although no longer considered to be the mainstream providers of medical care in Japan and viewed by many with some scepticism the traditional therapists do remain popular and offer a real and often effective alternative for many individuals when the services and treatment of 'western' medicine are of no avail. Many chronic problems or minor ailments (e.g. back problems, sore joints, stomach disorders) are relieved by regular sessions of massage, acupuncture, chiropractic, or herbal remedies. For many people the relief of pain and discomfort without drugs is what is most important, and they can get this relief from the traditional therapist, who is usually more concerned with the patient's total well-being than the modern doctor, whose focus is too often limited to the clinical disease alone. In cases where a 'cure' is an unrealistic expectation traditional therapies offer important psychological relief. In Japan today the traditional therapists appeal to quite distinct groups of patients; those individuals who have retained a more traditional approach to their health care, who are wary of the new medicine and who have probably been long-term clients of the acupuncturist or chiropractor; then a younger generation of modern Japanese who do not necessarily subscribe to the traditional beliefs about the nature and cause of illness but who are however sceptical about the efficacy of modern medicine and whose scepticism is moreover deepened by reports of malpractice, negligence, and the offhand manner of many doctors. Readers who wish to learn more about traditional therapies will find comprehensive and lucid discussion in the anthropological studies of Margaret Locke and Emiko Ohnuki Tierney.[14]

References

1 *Statistical Abstract of the USA 1984*, Washington D.C., United States Bureau of Census, 1985, p. 103.

2 These data obtained from Japanese language tables published by the Ministry of Health and Welfare, Tokyo.

3 Report on *Survey of Physicians, Dentists and Pharmacists* (Japanese), Statistics and Information Department, Ministry of Health and Welfare, Tokyo, 1986.

4 *Outline of Recent Japanese Policy on Health: The Background and Measures for Reform*, Ministry of Health and Welfare, Tokyo, November 1985, p. 24.

5 M.S. Bando, *Japanese Women Yesterday and Today*, Tokyo, Foreign Press Centre, 1986, pp. 16ff.

6 Pachinko parlours: pachinko is a form of pinball machine and players win small steel balls which can be exchanged for prizes. Although the prizes themselves have little value, they can be exchanged for cash at

nearby shops which specialize in this trade. With some 14 million devoted players in more than 10,000 parlours pachinko is a lucrative business.

7 *Trends and Policies of Health Services in Japan: Rationalising Medical Care Costs*, Japan International Corporation of Welfare Services (JICWELS), 1983, p. 13.

8 Wm E. Steslicke, *Doctors in Politics: The Political Life of the Japan Medical Association*, New York, Praeger, 1973, p. 37.

9 M. Hashimoto, 'Health services in Japan', in M.W. Raffel (ed.) *Comparative Health Systems*, Philadelphia, Penn. and London, Pennsylvania State University Press, 1984, p. 347.

10 There are 82 medical professional societies registered with the Japanese Association of Medical Sciences and all publish proceedings, journals, and newsletters; a further 150 organizations representing professionals in allied health care, hospital organizations, and others in health sciences are also known.

11 *Japan Times*, 12 June 1986.

12 W. Wetherall, 'To tell or not to tell – that is the question', *Far Eastern Economic Review*, 30 January 1986.

13 All statistics in the section on nursing services are taken from 'Statistical Data on Nursing Services in Japan, 1981' compiled under the supervision of the Nursing Division, Health Policy Bureau, Ministry of Health and Welfare, Tokyo.

14 M. Locke, *East Asian Medicine in Urban Japan*, Cambridge, Mass., University of California Press, 1980.
E. Ohnuki-Tierney, *Illness and Culture in Contemporary Japan*, Cambridge, Cambridge University Press, 1984.

Chapter nine

The future: Japan at a turning-point

In gathering together information and statistics about health care provisions in Japan we have tried to go beyond the usual bland presentation that might characterize official publications on the subject and we have consciously aimed to include our own assessments and criticism. In making his conclusions about health care in Japan today Masahira Anesaki undoubtedly brings into play greater knowledge of and insight into the workings of Japanese society and the Japanese mentality, an armamentarium of basic background information and sensitivity which might elude the short-term resident. But perhaps at the same time the relatively unbiased eye of the outsider (Margaret Powell) can see some things in sharper perspective.

An evaluation of the Japanese health care system – Margaret Powell

When we evaluate something we are necessarily making a value-judgement; in order to eliminate or at least reduce the impact of the subjective element we gather together and appraise facts and relevant information and apply explicit, universally accepted criteria to assess the subject. The concept of 'health' lacks a definition with world-wide validity and acceptance and the same goes for what health services should aim to be or achieve. And yet several criteria have been developed so that we can compare and evaluate different systems of care. The following assessment is structured around the criteria of equity, effectiveness, efficiency, quality, and satisfaction.

Equity

First let us consider equity which is defined at its simplest and most straightforward as 'justice' and 'fairness'. Attempts to produce a definition any more concrete than that invariably dissipate in a fog of different cultural and societal values, national ideas about the issue being notoriously flexible. Equity in health care should mean that provisions for health services are distributed within the community in a socially just manner, that some sectors of the community are not disadvantaged or missed out, and that payment and pricing mechanisms do not prevent any members of society from obtaining the care they need.

Over the past one hundred years Japan has certainly improved the distribution of medical care facilities and personnel and hence assured improvement in the public's access to services, an important dimension of equity in health care. As we saw in Chapter 6 Japan enjoys a high ratio of hospital beds per capita, one of the highest in the world, and on the whole the Japanese people do not encounter difficulties in gaining admission to hospital. The generous supply of physicians means that ambulatory medical care is likewise easy to obtain. Regional differences exist in the hospital bed to population and physician to population ratios; the city-dweller undoubtedly has greater choice than the country-dweller. But in absolute terms geographical obstacles are minor in nature. As far as we can ascertain the government has not evaluated such things as waiting times for admission to hospital or whether there are critical delays in obtaining treatment. As the majority of hospitals operate below maximum capacity these would not appear to be problems.

Since the introduction in 1961 of a universal compulsory insurance system which facilitates easy access to guaranteed and fairly standardized levels of service, the people of Japan are the beneficiaries of a system which ensures that their needs for medical care are well taken care of without any undue financial burden. Provisions for patients requiring long-term care or for people with mental handicap or mental illness are less satisfactory. Public assistance covers some gaps in insurance coverage, but many people do not take up their entitlement because of the real stigma attached to those who have to rely on state assistance rather than on their family.

We gave details in Chapter 5 of the complexities of the health insurance system and highlighted the present distribution of health care costs among public funds, the insurance carriers, and individuals. The health insurance system is universal and compulsory and from this perspective achieves equity. Nobody in Japan needs contemplate financial ruin in the event of illness; but the system is by no means standardized and hence may compromise the full achievement of equity. Depending on employment or residence, people are enrolled in different schemes whose premium contributions and benefits vary and there are clear advantages to membership in one scheme or another. Government has recognized that such differences are not in keeping with an equitable system and an important feature of present policy is the elimination of such discrepancies so that by the end of the century all insurance plans will confer the same level of benefits; cost-sharing at point of service will also be standardized.

It is certainly important to keep in mind the fact that official figures on health care expenditure in Japan do not capture the extent and volume of costs to the individual of 'extra-charge' services which are not included in insurance. The decision to have additional services is a personal one made after full details of the cost have been provided and those who do choose such extras are usually aware of the financial consequences of doing so. Equity in basic services is still maintained. The medical care provided does not in any case alter greatly from one grade of room to another as the doctors are on the staff of the hospital and treat all patients; they cannot be paid extra by the patient (at least not directly) in order to secure greater attention. The custom of giving presents to doctors is widespread but many hospitals, especially public ones, are taking concerted action to stamp out the practice.

There is otherwise little or no discrimination regarding the individual's access to and use of different components of the medical care delivery system. Patients in Japan have absolute freedom of choice of the type of service they can use when ill; indeed by comparison with most other countries, even those with similar fee-for-service arrangements, the choices are possibly too numerous and bewildering. Facilities are not linked to any specific insurance scheme and referrals are not required: the individual can go directly to a local practitioner, a clinic, or a large specialized hospital. In the absence of adequate consumer health education programmes people often consequently make poor or inappropriate selection and this consumer advantage is an important contributor to the inappropriate use and management of health services resources which brings us to the second criterion of evaluation: effectiveness.

Effectiveness

Effectiveness in health care concerns the relationship between inputs and health outcomes, whether the right resources are used properly to achieve planned and suitable outputs. It implies that a country is able to determine its specific goals for the inputs, process variables, and outcomes of health and medical services and can structure provisions in order to match assessed needs with available resources.

Evaluation of a health care system's performance has to rely at its simplest on reviewing statistics on mortality, especially infant mortality, and morbidity. The latter is as difficult to measure properly in Japan as everywhere and so we shall focus on mortality statistics. Japan's health status, as suggested by statistics on male and female life expectancy and infant mortality-rates, is better than it has ever been before and way ahead of all other developed countries. Starting from an exceptionally low base after the Second World War it has recorded much greater progress than other developed countries. The improvements in overall health status cannot however be attributed to medical and health provisions alone and even less to the way that they have been organized.

Other variables have operated in Japan as they have done elsewhere: developments in education, improved housing, better infrastructure, action for better environmental conditions, giant increases in prosperity widely spread through most of the population; in addition a traditional diet that has until recently conferred some important nutritional and hence health status advantages.

For a long time there was little official interest in evaluating the essential role and impact of the medical care system in the improvement of health status in the country; reviewing the development of health care resources in the face of such obvious progress was not deemed necessary. Indeed the official stance could probably be summed up as more is necessary and better. Only when it became obvious that the government was assuming a much larger and faster growing share of increasing health care costs did a policy giving any hint of consideration of the nature and deployment of resources in relation to outputs begin to emerge. Medical facilities have evolved in the country unfettered by government planning. With one or two notable exceptions the government has been content to keep a watchful eye from the sidelines on the provider-led development of services. Convinced that more medical facilities could be equated with better health care, the government fuelled this development in the 1960s by its pricing and financing mechanisms. The government's main contribution to facilities' development has been through support for the national medical centres and subsidies for services and health insurance administration. It has issued broad strategies and made recommendations about public health services. The latter programmes have been implemented by local authorities, who have autonomy to determine the nature and scope of their public health provisions. However local government health departments have little real authority or influence over the private sector operators in their area and cannot always determine the kind and quality of service which they provide in the community.

For longer than has been the case elsewhere the deployment of health care resources in Japan has been characterized by the separation and fragmentation of channels of service; public health programmes on the one hand and privately provided medical care on the other. Such provisions in the 1980s are ill-suited to the needs of a modern, highly-urbanized, dynamic, and yet ageing society.

The essential nature of Japan's medical care facilities has also affected the effectiveness of health care delivery. Without any real distinction among medical care facilities other than that of size, provisions have been skewed towards general acute hospital beds, although in many instances the term 'acute' is an inaccurate one. The practice of treating chronically ill, elderly, or disabled people in hospitals when they could be better cared for in facilities offering lower-intensity care has to be questioned. It is expensive to maintain such cases in the costly hospital setting but, in the absence to date of other kinds of facilities, it is the only approach available. Another serious consequence of the way resources have been organized is a disturbing lack of co-ordination between all the component parts; between the government and the private sector, among facilities and even, some would say, among different departments at the hospital level. For the patient there are often negative consequences for continuity and appropriateness of care.

The government has woken up to the ramifications of these structural weaknesses and hence its policy for the 1990s calls for greater delineation of functional roles and responsibilities among all facilities. The government has also started to scrutinize the nature and pattern of facilities' growth and is starting to promote the valuable concept of regional medical care planning, some thirty years, it might be added, after it was recommended as advisable. The prefectural health departments are now required to formulate medical services plans 'adapted to a region's actual conditions first and subsequently improve public and private medical care facilities'.[1] By comparison with the comprehensive and detailed service planning and resource allocation procedures used in the National Health Service for example, the Japanese initiative is primitive, but compared to what has gone before it represents a great conceptual leap forward into a brave new world!

The same lack of planning which has characterized facilities' development has been evident too for medical personnel development. There is a generous supply of doctors for the population as a whole: regional and geographical differentials are of minor consequence. Having achieved sufficiency in total numbers concern has gradually, and quite rightly, focused on whether the country has the right kinds of doctors and whether their training has been good enough and most fitting for changing population needs. Attention is going too to the pattern of extensive socialization by private practitioners and their lack of continuing education and training which have been detrimental to the promotion of primary health care in the community. The dominant role of the medical profession is also disturbing. Too many members of the medical profession remain reluctant to come to terms with the challenge of new requirements for health and medical care which demography and different disease patterns are imposing. Hanging on to considerable political power as it does the profession has ensured that doctors continue to dominate policy and decision-making in health care; in doing so they have furthermore managed to downplay, downgrade, and often ignore the actual and potential contribution of nurses and other allied health professionals. In pushing for primary health care the government is attempting to correct this imbalance but is still struggling to get real acceptance of the value of a teamwork approach in primary health care and for the moment the doctor holds the pivotal position. Within the hospital setting medical care teams function very well in Japan as hierarchial roles and status are accepted by all the participants. There are however resource implications for the continued dominance of doctors in other settings, where other professionals could be making just as effective a contribution to health care. The government meanwhile is sensibly employing the fee-reimbursement system in order to achieve its objectives of greater emphasis on primary health care and for private practitioners to function as family physicians rather than specialists. Hence preventive health care activities will be compensated, fees for referral to hospitals have been introduced in order to encourage some simple co-ordination of services; reimbursement of prescribed high-technology (and expensive) procedures will be made only to certain types of facilities; and the nature of clinical practice will be more closely scrutinized.

Efficiency

The third criterion of this evaluation, efficiency, has been a major preoccupation everywhere in recent years as countries have had to come to grips with the problem of providing more health services without at the same time imposing intolerable burdens on public expenditure.

To evaluate efficiency is to ask whether the health care system produces its intended results in the least costly way: to examine whether the financial investment secures optimum returns. Japan as we have seen was late to realize the implications of uncontrolled health care spending but having done so seems to have developed a fixation about cost containment without at the same time fully appreciating the need for setting some positive targets for her health care provisions.

Until recently Japan did not formally define the objectives of her health service. In coming down firmly on the side of cost-containment for the last two decades of the twentieth century the government is also now declaring its intentions about what the country's health and medical services should be achieving. The most recent policy statements note that 'Medical care expenditure must be rationalized and made more effective'.[2] The government has indicated that it will be taking a more active role than it has to date in monitoring costs and utilization of resources. Japan's health policy-makers are convinced that the existing *structure* of health care is right and that improved management will yield the desired surplus of benefits over costs. Proposals confirm that there will not be any radical departure from the current mode of services provision for the future.

In Chapter 5 we saw that Japan's official statistics on health care expenditure are deficient in that they encompass a limited number of resources. Official data not only do not accurately portray the real total cost of health and medical care to the country but also systematically under-report it. The official stance tends to give the impression that Japan operates a health care system that matches other areas of endeavour in efficiency and this is misleading.

In the absence of standard outcome variables for health care which can be used with cost data to assess efficiency it is customary to look at measures of the utilization of resources, to review throughput and performance indicators, and to study the cost of services provided from the point of view of those paying for them (the government, the individual, or the insurer) and to review the actions of the providers to ensure that they perform as efficiently as possible.

Hospitals everywhere are an expensive method of delivering health and medical care and the misuse of this resource amounts to inefficiency. Several factors associated with hospital usage in Japan suggest that this particular resource is not operated as efficiently as it might be. Japanese hospitals are a varied set of disparate facilities, the majority of them small and a considerable proportion of them too small to be able to reap the benefits of scale when it comes to running costs. In its entirety the hospital 'system' is not efficient since no single body has been in a position to oversee facilities development properly, to match needs at various levels with provisions, and thus to avoid a waste of resources. There is consequently unnecessary and costly duplication of facilities and services.

The hospitalization rate for the country is low by comparison with other developed countries, but it has been going up and there has been a disproportionate increase in the use of hospital out-patient departments for ambulatory health services. As Japan also has a generous supply of individual doctors this trend is disquieting. In the open access system it has also been difficult to control.

In Chapter 6 we saw that Japan records the longest average length of stay figures in the world and that the discrepancy between Japanese rates and other countries holds good even when the same disease categories are compared. While reduction in length of stay does not of itself automatically produce more efficient hospital services, prolongation of the patient stay in the hospital beyond the time when medical reasons justify it is undoubtedly a misuse and waste of resources. Few, if any, hospitals in Japan understand the positive values of such things as the planned short stay, the advantages which might be derived from out-patient surgery, five-day wards, and so forth either for reasons of efficiency or the patient's welfare. Only in the case of maternity (for normal labour and delivery) and abortions do Japan's length-of-stay figures approach prevailing world-wide norms. Neither of these is covered by the regular benefits of health insurance. A further inefficiency in the hospital system is revealed by the data on the number of cases per hospital bed: Japan treats seven cases per bed annually compared to the United Kingdom's twenty-five per bed, Sweden's sixteen per bed, New Zealand's twenty-three per bed, and Germany's sixteen per bed.[3]

In addition to the continuation of traditional inefficient medical practices and the fragmentation of service channels, the point-fee reimbursement system has adversely influenced efficiency: it offers no real incentive to hospitals to review or reconsider their policy and practice regarding patient admission and the length of patient stay. Individual physicians who run many hospitals are not fully aware of the impact of clinical practice and management on the overall management of the facility. Clinical judgement and freedom alone have governed the provision of services and with universal insurance and patient co-payment financial constraints on their practice have been few. Government policy will now force many hospitals to reconsider their management procedures and to look for ways of improving the organization of management of all activities and they are tackling the problems in a wide variety of ways. Smaller hospitals are joining together to buy supplies, pharmaceuticals, and equipment or to contract for housekeeping and domestic services in order to achieve the kind of economies of scale which as independent units they could not hope to do. Hospital administrators have generally played a secondary role to the medical staff in the hierarchy and their role has been confined to supervision of accounting, clerical, and domestic operations. The basic pattern of hospital administration is unlikely to change very much although there is a growing recognition of the need to have professionally trained hospital administrators who will work with greater managerial authority. The expanded use of management and clinical information systems and computerization will assist this trend. Municipally owned hospitals are even less efficient than the private ones but they have benefited in the past from government subsidies to bail them out.[4] With stricter government financing policy and the implementation of more rigorous monitoring and auditing procedures these facilities too are having to devote more attention to more efficient operations.

Quality and satisfaction

Finally let us consider the quality of health and medical care in Japan today: how satisfactorily do the providers of medical care perform, do they provide clinically advisable and suitable treatment which is in keeping with recognized professional standards? Do the providers deliver services which ensure patient satisfaction, important because it can enhance patient compliance with treatment and can contribute to the proper use of resources and services.

With regard to clinical competence, standards, and responsibilities, we suggested in Chapter 8 that there is some room for improvement in the basic education and training of the country's physicians. Medical practice is curatively oriented still and this bias is reflected in undergraduate medical education. Japan's doctors are not being trained to consider seriously anything other than what has gone before as being the successful route to good medical and health care. Standards of postgraduate education and training are remarkably varied and specialist training often commences too early in the doctor's career. Many specialists practise without the benefit of proper examination of their skills and knowledge. There are no formal mechanisms for monitoring the quality of care and appropriateness of the services they offer. The dual role of the individual practitioner – doctor and businessman – gives rise to some dubious medical practices and conflicts of interest. Too many doctors confuse intensity and quantity of treatment with quality of care and too many patients as a consequence leave their doctor's office none the wiser, but happy to be clutching a fistful of pills, too many of which are quite irrelevant.

Japan's hospitals lack formal systems for evaluating the nature and quality of the services they provide, government requirements for routine admissions and patient data being limited in scope and utilization. Japanese management in all areas of endeavour is characterized by the 'ie' or family style of organization; it is a style which is essentially paternalistic in nature, with a well-defined hierarchy for participants. Organizations expect and get total loyalty from their employees who are required to exercise self-control and self-inspection in the performance of their duties. In return the employees are accorded respect – they are assured as individuals of their intrinsic value to the organization and that the contribution they make to its achievements is indispensable. Bolstered by such reassurance and the group support which is a part and parcel of it, all professional and other employee groups in an organization work together in mutual confidence and trust to achieve the smooth operation of all services and activities. In the factory this management ethic results in the efficient production of goods, in health care beneficial services for patients. The latter too, knowing their position and relationship to the organization, feel assured that actions taken are in their best interests and tend to be compliant.

Japanese hospitals therefore set their own standards and expect their employees to conform to them for the sake of the organization as a whole; they are as a result reluctant to accept the value of or to employ formal inspection and evaluation procedures, especially those which might originate outside the organization. There has been very limited application of formal systems of evaluation of hospital management by government in the interests of improving efficiency. As for standards of clinical competence the medical profession has yet to be fully convinced of the value of such techniques as peer review and medical audit. The Japanese medical profession polices itself as it always has done; there is little likelihood of change for some time to come.

The government now picks up a major share of the total medical care bill for the country and should be cognizant of the advantages and disadvantages of the financing mechanisms which it employees for this purpose. The government has been reluctant to acknowledge that the point-fee reimbursement system suffers from a number of flaws which may compromise quality of care. The system is biased towards rewarding concrete items of service and does not differentiate between medical services provided by junior or senior medical staff. The system does not actively encourage thoughtful practice. 'Primary health care' is a favourite policy slogan and Japan's health care policy-makers evince the conviction that the 'family physician' is the panacea for all the problems associated with the provision of primary health care. Official thinking however does not go far enough; general practitioners alone cannot provide good primary health care but need to be supported by other health workers and other health and social services. Present health care financing mechanisms do not cover such services.

The health insurance system has not yet been used for measuring or controlling the quality of health care provided. We saw in Chapter 5 that the checking and monitoring systems of the Social Insurance Medical Care Fee Payment Fund have been utilized principally to control for fraud or financial mismanagement. The scheme could, with some modifications, become a valuable tool in a broader programme of quality control and assessment.

'The Ageing Society' is an issue, an obsession almost, which stalks through all areas of public policy in Japan in the 1980s as her policy-makers struggle to devise socially appropriate and financially tolerable programmes to care for the health and medical, pension, housing, and other needs of elderly people through to the twenty-first century. The challenge posed by the massive demographic shift to an ageing population is a leitmotiv informing all planning and discussion on health care provisions. The already considerable impact of the issue on the official collective psyche has been further reinforced by its coincidence with a downturn in the country's economic growth-rate and the subsequent restraint on public spending, never outstandingly large in Japan anyway. Important too has been the dispersion of social changes of a kind and scale which have not occurred before in Japan's transformation from a feudal to a modern society. The changes are not as deep as superficial appearances might immediately suggest and yet one can sense that Japan's policy-makers dismiss such changes too lightly and may be misinterpreting the evidence and indicators all around them.

In enforcing strict controls and limitations on public spending for health care as it proposes to do, the government may well endanger that equity in health and medical care which much of the policy between 1945 and the 1980s has been instrumental in achieving. The abolition of free health services and the reinstatement of cost-sharing for elderly people has certainly already compromised equity for at least one sector of the population. The government has recognized that present provisions of medical, health, and welfare services for elderly people are inadequate but proposals for the future do not inspire confidence that there will be great improvement. There are plans to develop 'intermediate facilities' for elderly people which will offer a combination of hospital medical care and residential home services. However, admission will be means-tested and monthly charges high: there will be a shortfall in the number of places and the numbers of people requiring them. Government policy to support, guide, and assist the private sector and to encourage local government bodies, private welfare organizations, volunteers, and private enterprise to join together to establish welfare services for elderly people may well exacerbate existing geographical imbalances in provisions.

Rather than adding to the multiplicity of facilities Japan's health care planners should be paying greater attention to the already abundant supply of hospital facilities and to reviewing the nature of the services they provide; to exploring possibilities which might arise from some restructuring of services in the smaller units and to making available requisite development funds. A priority should be the improvement of non-institutional health and welfare services for elderly people and the achievement of better co-ordination between all the components of the present medical care system.

Too many families are forced to place elderly relatives in hospitals when they would prefer to have them at home but in the absence of reliable support services their real choice is limited. The burden on many Japanese families for the care of elderly relatives, perhaps for as long as ten or twenty years, will increase and become a serious social problem. A new generation of young Japanese is maturing, one which has grown up in comfort and prosperity and which might not necessarily share the same outlook and sense of social and family responsibility as their parents.

In becoming a modern society Japan has shown a remarkable flair for selecting those elements of western science, technology, and culture which are advantageous to it, which can be easily integrated and hence successfully transformed into an entity which is then innately Japanese. At the same time Japan has succeeded in retaining a strong national identity and cultural integrity because, as Nakane suggests, 'the basic social grammar has hardly been affected' and the impact of all the imports while quite awesome has not disturbed, so far, the 'firm persistence of the basic nature and core of personal relationships and group dynamics'.[5]

Japan consciously and deliberately imported a foreign system of medical care some one hundred years ago and has since then turned it into something eminently suitable to Japan; it has met and successfully coped with new challenges posed by developments in medicine itself, by the innovations and inventions of technology, by shifts in the political background, by improvements in economic circumstances and by changes in the cultural environment. The country has fostered the evolution of a health care system which matches its cultural and social organization and ethic. For the most part the recipients of the system's output are happy and accept that provisions are organized as they are for their benefit. The outward appearance of the 'system' is deceptive; it is often unwieldy and cumbersome and forces the patient to be exactly that. But thoroughness, attention to individuals, and awareness of small, seemingly insignificant details is evident in Japanese health care, as indeed it is in all aspects of Japanese culture; in health care these characteristics combine to offer the reassurance which the patient needs and certainly override apparent failings in overall organization. In gradually modifying the organization and financing of the health care system Japan's success to date has depended largely on the achievement of consensus among all concerned, the service-providers, those paying for it, and those using it. There are certainly some grounds for concern that more radical and comprehensive kinds of change might be necessary if the present system is to be in a position to respond fully and to cope compassionately with the changes taking place in Japanese society and which will surely impinge on the health status of the people and their health care. I have no doubts that Japan has unique, admirable, and considerable resources to meet the challenges successfully.

Japanese health care at the turning-point or in crisis – Masahira Anesaki

In the two decades after the Second World War the health status of the Japanese people improved enormously and the health care delivery system likewise progressed and developed steadily into a modern system. I attribute the progress to the country's economic growth and political security and stability, which were aided by the guarantees provided under the Constitution of 1947, as follows:

> Article 25:
> 1. All people shall have the right to maintain the minimum standards of wholesome and cultured living.
> 2. In all spheres of life the State shall use its endeavours for the promotion and extension of social welfare and security, and of public health.

But as the end of the 1980s approaches I and many others feel that the Japanese health care system is facing a crisis, a crisis which has its roots in the early 1970s when radical changes in the country's economy resulting from the 'oil shock' of 1973 forced some radical rethinking of social welfare and health care policies by the government. Three salient factors contributed to changes in official health care policies:

1 Demography – a rapidly ageing population meant an increase in the prevalence of chronic degenerative diseases which were and remain costly to treat; it also meant that social security provisions for a larger proportion of the population had to be devised.
2 The increased pace of development in medical technology and the

greater use of the new, sophisticated, and expensive technology in medical care.

3 Low economic growth and a reduction in government revenues from tax and health-related insurance.

The first two factors caused government expenditure to rise, whereas the third factor reduced its available income. Finding it impossible to increase available funds for health care expenditure, the government in these circumstances developed a health care policy, the main plank of which has been cost-containment. Key events and dates in this policy have been as follows:

1973: The beginning as well as the end of the social welfare epoch in Japan (introduction of free medical care for elderly people, reduction in the amount of co-payment by dependants, the introduction of a maximum monthly co-payment, the beginning of low economic growth-rates for the country).

1981: The appointment of the Second Emergency Administrative Reform Council.

1982: Resignation of Dr Taro Takemi, president of the Japan Medical Association for the previous twenty-five years.

1983: Reintroduction of co-payment of medical care for elderly people.

1984: Introduction of 10 per cent co-payment at point of service for insurees.

1985: Primary reform of the Medical Service Law (introduced regional medical planning to limit the numbers of hospital beds, and system for inspection and supervision of medical facilities).

1986: Plan to reduce numbers of national hospitals and sanatoria or for privatization of such facilities. Reports of government committees on Demand for Physicians and on the Family Physician.

1987: Interim report on the Nation's General Medical Policy. Reform of the Elderly People's Health Act on the introduction of specialized health facilities for elderly people.

1988: Proposals on health and welfare policies by junior civil servants of the Ministry of Health and Welfare.

Japan did not introduce medical care cost-containment measures as early perhaps as it should have done; partly because of government optimism about the state of the overall economy and partly because of immense political pressure from the Japan Medical Association under the leadership of a powerful and dominant president, Dr Taro

Takemi. Real efforts to contain the growth in medical care expenditure really got under way only in the early 1980s. After the Second Administrative Reform Council was established and once Dr Takemi had resigned from office the government was able to accelerate its policies to control health care spending.

Early measures, implemented in the first half of the 1980s, were designed to operate through the health insurance schemes and encompassed first the introduction and then the increase of patient co-payment at point of service; the reduction in the standard wholesale price of drugs, and stricter monitoring and control of medical and hospital bills submitted to the government for reimbursement. Subsequent measures to control growth in health care costs have begun to tackle structural aspects of the Japanese health care system. These have included attempts to modify health and welfare services delivery systems and the introduction of some formalized services planning mechanisms.

Effects and prospects of the cost-containment policy

As we saw in Chapter 5, Japan's national health expenditure increased by more than 10 per cent per annum for twenty years until the late 1970s, with a record 36.2 per cent increase in 1974. The rate of the annual increase certainly dropped in the early 1980s and the changes introduced in the health insurance schemes can be properly credited with achieving some of the drop. But since 1985 total national medical care expenditure is again on the increase and government attempts to control the annual rate of growth in this increase have signally failed. This demonstrates that control of Japan's health care expenditures cannot be achieved by simply tinkering with the details of the health insurance system, because to do so will result in only short-term or limited reductions in overall expenditure. Real and long-term cost-containment will be gained only via radical changes in the health care and social welfare services delivery system itself; this can be illustrated by an experimental project which was set up in the village of Sawauchi in northern Japan. In this community health care project, free ambulatory medical care for elderly people was introduced as far back as 1960, some thirteen years before the government introduced its nation-wide scheme. In addition free medical care was offered for infants aged 1 year and under, home visits were provided by doctors and public health nurses; health education programmes were devised and delivered in the community and free preventive health check-ups were provided. In addition there was some reform of housing and other social services in the community. The project was carefully monitored and by the end of the 1970s there had been a striking change in patterns of service usage and cost of health care provision. Particularly striking was the change from low medical consultation rates coupled with high medical care costs to a much higher consultation rate, coupled with a low medical care cost. Administrators and health care personnel worked together to improve access to health care services: records have shown remarkable improvements in basic health status indices in the community and a reduction in per capita medical care costs. It still remains unclear whether the Sawauchi village's experience is an exceptional or isolated one or if it could be replicated on a nation-wide basis. Present official views respect the experiment but the government will not sponsor any larger-scale programmes of a similar nature.

Japan continues to enjoy relatively good economic performance and the ratio of health care expenditure for size of population remains extremely low by international standards. Many observers therefore might, with some justification, question Japan's concern to contain growth in medical care costs and the development of such strict measures designed to achieve this end. It is true that Japan has a huge trade surplus, the income from which has been channelled to investments in overseas securities and real estate and that Japan is currently the world's largest creditor nation. But the government's income plus domestic demand have not grown so much. Moreover health, education, and welfare programmes are typically the last areas to benefit from the country's overall economic prosperity. It seems likely therefore that the government will not only maintain but also strengthen its medical care cost-containment policies, insisting on 'self-help' and privatization of selected services in order to save government expenditure.

Cost-containment policies focused initially on changes in the health insurance schemes but more recently attention has turned to the nature of the health care delivery system. And yet the government has acknowledged that there are some fundamental limitations to the achievement of its objectives caused by the nature of the system itself, but which it is not yet prepared to alter.[6] The government has no plans to change the existing free access which the public enjoys to the largely uncontrolled network of small individually owned medical facilities; so duplication of services will continue to contribute to unnecessary costs. Equally it has decided against allowing the introduction of American-style joint stock company hospital systems. The health insurance system will also remain as it is presently organized.

In a country which has wholeheartedly accepted in so many areas the benefits of modern science and technology and where modern medical equipment is widely used and favoured, there remains a singular area of controversy and debate. Organ transplantation and the application of genetic engineering have raised extremely difficult ethical problems for Japan. The traditional Japanese sense of death is characterized by the notion that a person dies only when the heart stops beating and to remove any organ from a person who has been declared brain dead damages the wholeness of the body. In January 1988 the Japan Medical Association, after some twenty years of on-and-off debate of the issue, declared that brain death instead of cessation of the heart could be acknowledged as the death of the person, thus opening the way to heart transplants and broadening the way to transplants of other organs. The Japanese public still harbours mixed feelings about the issue of brain death versus heart death and opposition to organ transplantation remains strong. The Japanese medical profession is still reluctant therefore to develop further the application of this particular form of medical treatment on a broad scale.

This book is the result of a joint effort by two authors, one is an outsider, the other an insider of Japan; taking advantage of characteristics of the background of both of us we have tried to give a comprehensive picture of Japan's health care rather than a deep analysis of specific aspects of it: this we have left to other authors. The two main objectives of the book have been to help contribute to international comparisons of health care systems and to further an understanding of Japan. Both authors sincerely hope that these objectives have been met.

References

1 Ministry of Health and Welfare, *Outline of Recent Japanese Policy on Health: The Background and Measures for Reform*, Tokyo, OECD, November 1985, p. 22.
2 ibid., p. 18.
3 OECD, *Measuring Health Care 1960–1983: Expenditure, Costs and Performance*, Social Policy Studies 2, Paris, OECD, 1985, p. 115.
4 K. Naito, 'Efficient hospital management', *Hospitals*, 2, July 1983, pp. 45–8.
5 C. Nakane, *Japanese Society*, Tokyo, C.E. Tuttle, 1984; London, Weidenfeld & Nicolson, 1970, pp. 153–4.
6 Ministry of Health and Welfare, *Interim Report of the Headquarters of the General Policies on the Nation's Medical Care*, 26 June 1987; *Report of the Commission on the Modernization and Stabilization of Medical Care Facilities*, 24 September 1987.

Appendix 1 Map of Japan

1. Hokkaido (Sapporo)
2. Aomori (Aomori)
3. Iwate (Morioka)
4. Miyagi (Sendai)
5. Akita (Akita)
6. Yamagata (Yamagata)
7. Fukushima (Fukushima)
8. Ibaraki (Mito)
9. Tochigi (Utsunomiya)
10. Saitama (Urawa)
11. Gumma (Maebashi)
12. Chiba (Chiba)
13. Tokyo (Tokyo)
14. Kanagawa (Yokohama)
15. Niigata (Niigata)
16. Toyama (Toyama)
17. Ishikawa (Kanazawa)
18. Fukui (Fukui)
19. Yamanashi (Kofu)
20. Nagano (Nagano)
21. Gifu (Gifu)
22. Shizuoka (Shizuoka)
23. Aichi (Nagoya)
24. Mie (Tsu)
25. Shiga (Otsu)
26. Kyoto (Kyoto)
27. Osaka (Osaka)
28. Hyogo (Kobe)
29. Nara (Nara)

Japan is made up of four main islands – Hokkaido, Honshu, Shikoku and Kyushu from north to south. The total land area is 377,765 sq. km.

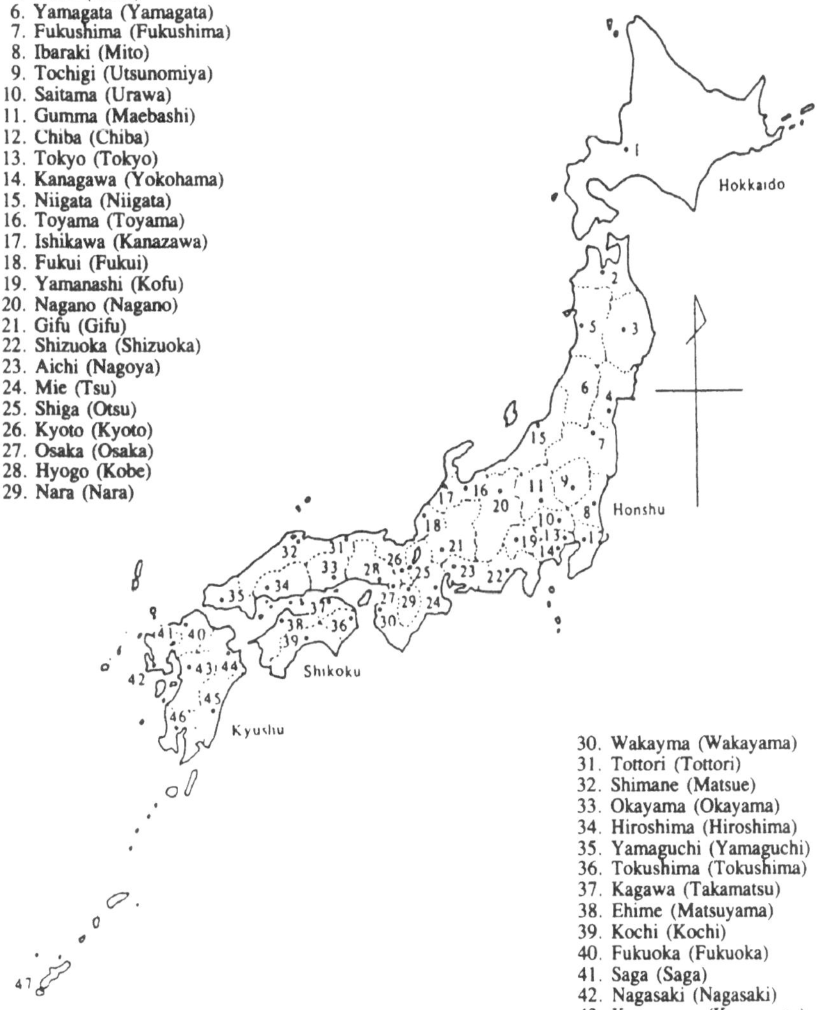

30. Wakayma (Wakayama)
31. Tottori (Tottori)
32. Shimane (Matsue)
33. Okayama (Okayama)
34. Hiroshima (Hiroshima)
35. Yamaguchi (Yamaguchi)
36. Tokushima (Tokushima)
37. Kagawa (Takamatsu)
38. Ehime (Matsuyama)
39. Kochi (Kochi)
40. Fukuoka (Fukuoka)
41. Saga (Saga)
42. Nagasaki (Nagasaki)
43. Kumamoto (Kumamoto)
44. Oita (Oita)
45. Miyazaki (Miyazaki)
46. Kagoshima (Kagoshima)
47. Okinawa (Naha)

Appendix 2 Chronology

660 BC	Traditional date of accession of first Emperor, Jimmu
710–784	Nara Period
794–866	Heian Period
866–1160	Fujiwara Period
1160–1333	Kamakura Period
1336–1392	Yoshino Period
1338–1573	Ashikaga (Muromachi) Period
1600–1867	Tokugawa Period
1868–1912	Meiji Period
1912–1926	Taisho Period
1926–1989	Showa Period
1989–	Heisei Period

Appendix 3 Exchange rates 1955–86

All financial data in the text are shown in yen. The following table gives the US dollar/yen and pound sterling/yen exchange rates for selected dates.

Date	*US$/Yen*	*£/Yen*
31 December 1955	359.67	1008
31 December 1960	358.20	
31 December 1965	360.99	
31 December 1970	357.45	308
31 December 1975	239.85	
31 December 1980	249.70	359.44
31 December 1981	220.10	421.30
31 December 1982	235.75	382.40
31 December 1983	233.50	332.40
30 June 1984	237.95	322.10
31 December 1984	251.05	292.20
30 June 1985	248.40	325.40
31 December 1985	200.35	288.70
30 June 1986	165.00	252.40

Appendix 4 Ownership of hospital facilities, 1986

National	Ministry of Health and Welfare; Ministry of Education: national university of teaching hospitals Ministry of Health and Welfare: national hospitals and national specialist centres Ministry of Labour: labour accident hospitals
Public	Local government: prefectural municipal Japan Red Cross Saisekai-Philanthropic Organization founded in nineteenth century Hokkaido Social Workers Association Federation of Farmers Associations Federation of National Health Insurance Societies
Private	Social Insurance Bodies: Federation of Social Insurance Societies Employees Pension Welfare Corporation Seamen's Insurance Society Federation of Health Insurance Societies National Health Insurance Societies Medical juridical persons Individuals Non-profit juridical persons School organizations Companies: Japan National Railways Others Salt and Tobacco Monopoly

Appendix 5 Medical schools in Japan, 1986

National institutions	Date established
Nagasaki University, School of Medicine	1857
University of Tokyo, Faculty of Medicine	1858
Osaka University, Faculty of Medicine	1869
Kumamoto University, Faculty of Medicine	1871
Tohoku University, Faculty of Medicine	1872
Nagoya University, School of Medicine	1873
Chiba University, School of Medicine	1876
Okayama University, School of Medicine	1879
Kanazawa Ubiversity, School of Medicine	1879
Kyoto University, Faculty of Medicine	1899
Kyushu University, Faculty of Medicine	1903
Hokkaido University, Faculty of Medicine	1919
Niigata University, School of Medicine	1922
Kagoshima University, School of Medicine	1942
Gunma University, School of Medicine	1943
Mie University, Faculty of Medicine	1943
Tokyo Medical and Dental University	1944
Hirosaki University, Faculty of Medicine	1944
Shinshu University, Faculty of Medicine	1944
Gifu University, School of Medicine	1944
Kobe University, Faculty of Medicine	1944
Tottori University, School of Medicine	1945
Hiroshima University, School of Medicine	1945
University of Tokushima, School of Medicine	1945
Yamaguchi University, School of Medicine	1949
Akita University, School of Medicine	1970
Asahikawa Medical College	1973
Yamagata University, School of Medicine	1973
The University of Tsukuba, School of Medicine	1973
Ehime University, School of Medicine	1973
National Defence Medical College	1973

Shiga Medical University	1974
Hamamatsu Medical College	1974
Miyazaki Medical College	1974
Shimane Medical University	1974
Toyama Medical and Pharmaceutical University	1975
Ohita Medical College	1976
Saga Medical College	1976
Kochi Medical College	1976
Yamanashi Medical College	1978
Fukui Medical College	1978
Kagawa Medical College	1978
University of Ryukyus, School of Medicine	1979

Total: forty-three facilities

Municipal institutions

Kyoto Prefectural University of Medicine	1875
Ngoya City University, School of Medicine	1943
Sapporo Medical College	1944
Fukushima Medical College	1944
Yokohama Municipal University, School of Medicine	1944
Osaka City University, School of Medicine	1944
Nara Medical College	1945
Wakayama Prefectural Medical College	1945

Total: eight facilities

Private institutions

Jikei University, School of Medicine	1880
Tokyo Women's Medical College	1912
Nippon Medical School	1915
Tokyo University, School of Medicine	1918
Keio University, School of Medicine	1920
Toho University, School of Medicine	1925
Nihon University, School of Medicine	1925
Osaka Medical College	1927
Showa University, School of Medicine	1928
Kansai Medical School	1928
Kurume University, School of Medicine	1928
Iwate Medical University	1928
Juntendo University, School of Medicine	1943
Fujita-Gakuen School of Medicine and Medical Technology	1966

Kyorin University, School of Medicine	1970
Kitasato University, School of Medicine	1970
Kawasaki Medical College	1970
St Marianna University, School of Medicine	1971
Aichi Medical University	1971
Teikyo University, School of Medicine	1971
Hyogo Medical College	1971
Dokkyo University, Faculty of Medicine	1972
Jichi Medical School	1972
Saitama Medical College	1972
Fukuoka University, Faculty of Medicine	1972
Kanazawa Medical University	1972
Kinki University, Faculty of Medicine	1974
Tokai University, School of Medicine	1974
Sangyo Medical College	1977

Total: twenty-nine facilities

Appendix 6 Professional organizations and research institutions

Below is a select list of the principal organizations and research institutions in health care in Japan.

1 Cancer Institute (Japan Foundation for Cancer Research),
37-1 Kami Ikebukuro 1 Chome,
Toshima Ku,
Tokyo 170
Tel: (03) 918-0111

2 Institute of Medical Science (University of Tokyo),
4-6-1 Shiroganedai,
Minato Ku,
Tokyo 108
Tel: (03) 443-8111

3 National Cancer Centre,
5-1-1 Tsukiji,
Chuo Ku,
Tokyo 104
Tel: (03) 542-2511

4 National Institute for Leprosy Research,
4-2-1 Aoba-Cho,
Higashi Murayama
T189
Tel: (0423) 91-8211

5 National Institute of Health,
2-10-35 Kamiosaki,
Shinagawa Ku,
Tokyo 141
Tel: (03) 444-2181

6 National Institute of Hospital Administration,
1-21-13 Toyama,
Shinjuku Ku,
Tokyo 162
Tel: (03) 203-5327

7 National Institute of Hygienic Science,
1-18-1 Kamiyoga,
Setagaya Ku,
Tokyo 158
Tel: (03) 700-1141
8 National Institute of Nutrition,
1-23-1 Toyama,
Shinjuku Ku,
Tokyo 162
Tel: (03) 203-5721
9 Research Institute, Japan Anti TB Association,
3-1-24 Matsuyama,
Kiyose,
T180-04
Tel: (0424) 93-5711
10 Tokyo Metropolitan Research Laboratory of Public Health,
3-24-1 Hyakunin Cho,
Shinjuku Ku,
Tokyo 160
Tel: (03) 363-3231
11 Japan Dental Associations,
3-16 Hayabusa Cho,
Chiyoda Ku,
Tokyo 102
Tel: (03) 262-1141
12 Japan Medical Association,
2-5 Kanda Surugadai,
Chiyoda Ku,
Tokyo 101
Tel: (03) 291-2121
13 Japan Pharmaceutical Association,
2-12-15 Shibuya,
Shibuya Ku,
Tokyo 150
Tel: (03) 406-1171
14 Japan Nutrition Association,
Rakucho Building,
2-1 Yurakacho 2 Chome,
Chiyoda Ku,
Tokyo 100

15 Japanese Nursing Association,
5-8-2 Jingumae,
Shibuya Ku,
Tokyo 150
Tel: (03) 400-8331

16 Japan Hospital Association,
2-14 Kojimachi,
Chiyoda Ku,
Tokyo 102
Tel: (03) 265-0077

17 Japanese Red Cross Society,
1-1-3 Shiba Daimon,
Minato Ku,
Tokyo 105
Tel: (03) 438-1311

18 Medical Instruments Society of Japan,
3-3915 Hongo,
Bunkyo Ku,
Tokyo 113
Tel: (03) 813-1062

19 Japan Association of Medical Equipment Industry,
Eikoo Hike Hongo Building,
3-32-6 Hongo,
Bunkyo Ku,
Tokyo 113
Tel: (03) 816-5575

20 Federation of Pharmaceutical Manufacturers Association of Japan,
Tokyo Yakugyo Kaikan Building,
9 Nihonbashi Hon-Cho, 2 Chome,
Chuo Ku,
Tokyo 103
Tel: (03) 270-0581

21 Japan Chiropractic College,
Higashi Ginza Building, 6th Floor,
8-18-4 Ginza,
Tokyo 104
Tel: (03) 545-5768

22 Japan Public Health Association,
1-29-8 Shinjuku,
Shinjuku Ku,
Tokyo 160
Tel: (03) 352-4281

23 National Council of Social Welfare,
3-3-4 Kasumigaseki,
Chiyoda Ku,
Tokyo 100
Tel: (03) 581-7851

24 The Japanese Society of Health and Medical Sociology,
c/o Department of Sociology,
Japan Red Cross University,
4-1-3 Hiroo,
Shibuyaku,
Tokyo 150
Tel: (03) 409-0875

25 The Japan Research Institute on Child Welfare Inc.,
4-2-12 Kudan Minami,
Chiyoda Ku,
Tokyo 102
Tel: (03) 234-6951

26 Japanese Organization for International Co-operation in Family Planning Inc.,
Hoken Kaikan Bekkan,
1-1 Ichigaya, Sadohara Cho,
Shinjuku Ku,
Tokyo 162
Tel: (03) 268-5875

A further eighty-five organizations representing medical and scientific and other professional groups in the health sciences are members of the Japanese Association of Medical Sciences:

2-5 Kanda Surugadai,
Chiyoda Ku,
Tokyo 101
Tel: (03) 291-2121

The Association has a detailed listing of the names and addresses of members in Japanese. Readers interested in obtaining information from this organization or the groups noted above may try writing to them directly.

Bibliography

This is divided into three sections. The first section contains a selection of some of the more accessible and yet useful works on Japan for those readers who would like to expand their general reading on the country. The second section lists those works which deal specifically with health and medical care in Japan. The third section contains a short selection of books and other publications dealing with the health sciences.

General reading

Barr, P., *The Coming of the Barbarians: A Story of Western Settlement in Japan, 1853–1870*, Tokyo, C.E. Tuttle, 1967.

Beasley, W.G. (ed.), *Modern Japan: Aspects of History, Literature and Society*, Tokyo, C.E. Tuttle, 1976, London, Allen & Unwin, 1975.

Benedict, R., *The Chrysanthemum and the Sword – Patterns of Japanese Culture*, Tokyo, C.E. Tuttle, 1946.

Christopher, R.C., *The Japanese Mind*, New York, Fawcett Columbine, 1983.

Doi, T., *The Anatomy of Dependence*, trans. J. Bester, 3rd edn, Tokyo, New York, San Francisco, Kodansha International, 1984.

Dore, R.P., *Shinohata: A Portrait of a Japanese Village*, New York, Pantheon, 1978.

Drummond, R.H.A., *A History of Christianity in Japan*, Grand Rapids, Michigan, Wm B. Erdmans Publishing, 1971.

Fraser, M.C., *A Diplomat's Wife in Japan*, ed. H. Cortazzi, Tokyo, Weatherhill, 1982.

Fukutake, T. *The Japanese Social Structure*, trans. R.P. Dore, Tokyo, University of Tokyo Press, 1982.

Hall, J.W., *Japan from Prehistory to Modern Times*, New York, Dell Publishing, 1970.

Hall, J.W. and Beasley, R.K., *Twelve Doors to Japan*, New York, McGraw-Hill, 1965.

Livingstone, J., Moore, J., and Oldfeather, F. (eds), *The Japan Reader, Vol. I, Imperial Japan 1800–1945* and *Vol. II, Postwar Japan, 1945–the*

Present, New York, Random House and Harmondsworth, Penguin, 1973.
MacDonald, D., *A Geography of Modern Japan*, Woodchurch, Paul Norbury Publications, 1985.
Nakane, C., *Japanese Society*, Tokyo, C.E. Tuttle, 1984; London, Weidenfeld & Nicolson, 1970.
Popham, P., *Tokyo, the City at the End of the World*, Tokyo, Kodansha International, 1985.
Rankle, S.F., *An Introduction to Japanese History*, Tokyo, International Society for Educational Information Press Inc. with Mainichi Newspapers, 1956.
Reischauer, E.O., *Japan: The Story of a Nation*, Tokyo, C.E. Tuttle, 1974.
Shiratori, R. (ed.), *Japan in the 1980s*, Tokyo, Kodansha International, 1982; New York, Harper & Row, 1982.
Storry, R., *A History of Modern Japan*, Harmondsworth, Penguin, 1960, revised edn, 1983.
Taylor, J., *Shadows of the Rising Sun: A Critical View of the Japanese Miracle*, Tokyo, C.E. Tuttle, 1983.

Health and medical care

Atoh, M., 'Changes in fertility and fertility control behaviour', in M. Muramatsu and T. Katagiri (eds), *Readings on Population and Family Planning in Japan*, Tokyo, Japanese Organization for International Co-operation in Family Planning, Inc., 1985.
Baelz, E., *Awakening Japan: The Diary of a German Doctor*, Bloomington, Indiana, Indiana University Press, 1974.
Bando, M., *Japanese Women, Yesterday and Today*, Tokyo, Foreign Press Centre, 1986.
Chester, T. and Ichien, M., 'Health care in Japan – its development, structure and problems', *Three Banks Review*, 137, March 1983.
Collick, M., 'A different society', in *Inside Japan*, London, BBC, 1981.
Cortazzi, H., *Dr Willis in Japan, 1862–1877: A British Medical Pioneer*, London, Athlone Press, 1985.
Coleman, S., *Family Planning in Contemporary Japanese Society: Traditional Birth Control in a Modern Urban Culture*, Princeton, NJ, Princeton University Press, 1983.
Foreign Press Centre, *Administrative Reform in Japan*, Tokyo, Foreign Press Centre, 1984.
——— *The Japanese Family*, Reference Reading Series 9, Tokyo, 1982.
——— *Japan's Rapidly Aging Population*, Reference Reading Series 9, Tokyo, 1982.
Hashimoto, M., 'National health administration in Japan', *Bulletin of the Institute of Public Health*, 30, 1, Tokyo, 1981.
——— 'Health services in Japan', in M.W. Raffel (ed.), *Comparative Health Systems*, Philadelphia, Penn. and London, Pennsylvania State University Press, 1984.
Hashimoto, M., Hagishima, T., Muraura, K., and Shimada, K., 'Study on the role of health centres in health care for the aged', *Bulletin of the*

Institute of Public Health, 30, 1, Tokyo, 1981.
Health and Welfare Services in Japan, 1985, Ministry of Health and Welfare, Japan International Corporation of Welfare Services (JICWELS), Tokyo, 1986.
Health and Welfare Statistics in Japan, 1985, Health and Welfare Statistics Association, Tokyo, 1985.
Hinohara, S., Hinohara, M., and Hirofumi, T., 'A study on the evaluation of health and lifestyle habits in a rural area of Japan', *Medical Informatics*, 7, 3, 229–34, 1982.
Ichijo, K. and Kiikuni, K., 'Health services in Japan', *Japan=Hospitals*, 1, 30 July 1982, 2-30.
Ikegami, N., 'The Japanese health system – another success story?', *Hospital and Health Services Review*, 261–4, November 1984.
Ikegami, N. and Goldsmith, S.B., 'The Japanese health service – an overview', *Journal of Ambulatory Care*, 78–85, November 1982.
Japan in the Year 2000: Preparing Japan for the Age of Internationalisation, the Aging Society and Maturity, Long-Term Outlook Committee, Economic Council, Economic Planning Agency, Tokyo, Japan Times Ltd, 1983.
Japanese Organization for International Co-operation in Family Planning, Inc., *A Bird's Eye View of Population and Family Planning in Japan*, Tokyo, 1982.
——— *A Twenty Year History of Maternal and Child Health Centers*, Document Series 7, Tokyo, 1982.
Katabami, J., Kaneko, I., Oda, S., and Mugitani, M., 'A survey of physician activities', *Bulletin of the Institute of Public Health*, 30, 1, 1981.
Kato, M., 'Self-destruction in Japan: A cross-cultural epidemiological analysis of suicide', in T.S. Lebra and W.P. Lebra (eds), *Japanese Culture and Behaviour: Selected Readings*, Honolulu, Hawaii, University of Hawaii Press, 1974.
Kawakami, T., 'The situation of medical care in Japan and its problems', in M. Perlman (ed.), *Economics of Health and Medical Care*, Macmillan, 1974.
Kiikuni, K., 'Quality assurance in Japanese hospitals', *World Hospitals*, XVIII, 2, May 1982.
Kran, K., 'Internationalisation of Japan's pharmaceutical regulations', *American Chamber of Commerce Journal*, 23, 5, May 1986.
Keizai Koho Center, *Economic Views from Japan*, Selections from Economic Eye, Japan Institute for Social and Economic Affairs, Tokyo, 1986.
McCaffrey, D., 'Pills and potions', *Tokyo Journal*, January 1986.
McKnight, S., 'Japan's pharmaceutical industry no longer soaring', in M.A. Samson (ed.), *American Chamber of Commerce Journal*, Report 45a, November 1985.
Ministry of Health and Welfare, *Statistical Data on Nursing Service in Japan, 1984*, compiled under supervision of Nursing Division, Health Policy Bureau, Tokyo, 1984.

——— *Outline of Recent Japanese Policy on Health: The Background and Measures for Reform*, Tokyo, OECD, November 1985.
Morohashi, Y., 'The Japanese health insurance system', *Japan=Hospitals*, 3, 7–13, July 1984.
Muramatsu, M. and Katagiri, T. (eds) *Basic Readings on Population and Family Planning in Japan*, Tokyo, Japanese Organization for International Co-operation in Family Planning, Inc., 1985.
National Federation of Health Insurance Societies, *Situations and Trends of Medical Insurance and Medical Supply in Japan, 1985*, Tokyo, 1985.
Nikkei Industry Research Institute, *Japanese Health Care System*, Nikkei High Tech Report, Tokyo, 9 December 1985.
Ohmura, J., 'Overview of Japanese health insurance', *Japan=Hospitals*, 2, 17–31, July 1983.
Ohtani, F., *One Hundred Years of Health Progress in Japan*, International Medical Society of Japan, Tokyo, 1977.
——— *Medical and Public Health Services in Japan*, Proceedings of the First Asian Seminar on Health and Medical Sociology, Japanese Society of Health and Medical Sociology, Tokyo, 1981.
Social Insurance Agency, *Outline of Social Insurance in Japan, 1984*, Japan International Social Security Association, Tokyo, 1985.
Steslicke, W., *Doctors in Politics: The Political Life of the Japan Medical Association*, New York, Praeger, 1973.
Toufexis, A. and Ishikawa, Y., 'Prognosis: steady improvement', *Time Magazine*, 1 August 1983.
Wagatsuma, T., 'Induced abortion in Japan', in Y. Muramatsu and T. Katagiri (eds), *Basic Readings on Population and Family Planning in Japan*, Japanese Organization for International Co-operation in Family Planning, Inc., Tokyo, 1985.
Wakatsuki, T., 'Japanese rural hospitals and district health care activities', *Japan=Hospitals*, 3, 35–41, July 1984.
Weatherall, W., 'To tell or not to tell – that is the question', *Far Eastern Economic Review*, 34–6, 30 January 1986.
Yamamoto, M., 'Health of the people: how important are the decision-makers?', *International Journal of Health Education*, 20, 279–81, 1977.
——— 'Primary health care and health education in Japan', *Social Science and Medicine*, 17, 19, 141–3, 1983.

Health services

Abel-Smith, B., *Value for Money in Health Services*, London, Heinemann Educational Books, 1979.
Acheson, R.M., 'The definition and identification of need for health care', *Journal of Epidemiology and Community Health*, 32, 10–15, 1978.
Allsop, J., *Health Policy and the National Health Service*, London, Longman, 1984.
Altenstetter, C., 'Hospital planning in France and the Federal Republic of Germany', *Health, Politics, Policy and Law*, 5, 2, 309–32, 1980.

Bates, E., *Health Systems and Public Scrutiny: Australia, Britain and the United States*, London, Croom Helm, 1983.
Bevan, G., Copeman, H., Perrin, J., and Rosser, R., *Health Care Priorities and Management*, London, Croom Helm, 1980.
Bryant, J.H., 'Principles of justice as a basis for conceptualising a health care system', *International Journal of Health Services*, 7, 4, 707–19, 1977.
Butler, J.R. and Vaile, M.S.B., *Health and Health Services: An Introduction to Health Care in Britain*, London, Routledge & Kegan Paul, 1984.
Chaplin, N.W. (ed.), *Health Care in the United Kingdom: Its Organisation and Management*, Institute of Health Service Administrators, London, Kluwer Medical, 1982.
Chubb, P., Haywood, S., and Torrens, P., *Managing the Mixed Economy of Health*, Occasional Paper 42, University of Birmingham, Health Services Management Centre, 1982.
Creasey, W., *Diet and Cancer*, Pennsylvania, Lea & Febiger, 1985.
Dubos, R., *Man, Medicine and Environment*, Harmondsworth, Penguin, 1970.
Ham, C., *Health Policy in Britain*, London, Macmillan, 1982.
Klein, R., *The Politics of the NHS*, London, Longman, 1983.
LeGrand, J. and Robinson, R., *The Economics of Social Problems*, London, Macmillan, 1976.
Maxwell, R., *International Comparisons of Health Needs and Services*, King's Fund Project Paper RC 9, 1980.
OECD, *Measuring Health Care 1960–1983: Expenditure, Costs and Performance*, Social Policy Studies 2, Paris, OECD, 1985.
Raffel, M.W., *Comparative Health Systems: Descriptive Analyses of Fourteen National Health Systems*, Philadelphia, Penn. and London, Pennsylvania State University Press, 1984.
Roemer, M.I., *Health Care Systems in World Perspective*, Ann Arbor, Mich., Health Administration Press, 1976.
——— *Comparative National Policies on Health Care*, New York, Marcel Dekker, 1977.
Rosenthal, G. and Fox, D.M., 'A right to what? Towards adequate minimum standards of personal health services', *Millbank Memorial Fund Quarterly/Health and Society*, 56, 1, 1–21, 1978.
Simanis, J.G., *National Health Systems in Eight Countries*, Washington, DC, DHEW Publications, 1975.
Sorkin, A.L., *Health Economics: An Introduction*, Lexington, Mass., Heath Lexington Books, 1975.
Taylor, R., *Medicine Out of Control – The Anatomy of a Malignant Technology*, Melbourne, Sun Books, 1979.
Townsend, P. and Davidson, N., *Inequalities in Health: The Black Report*, Harmondsworth, Penguin, 1982.
WHO, *Health Economics*, WHO Public Health Reader, 64, Geneva and New York, July 1976.
Williams, A., *Health Service Objectives*, King's Fund Project Paper 10, London, 1980.

Index